HUMAN AGAIN

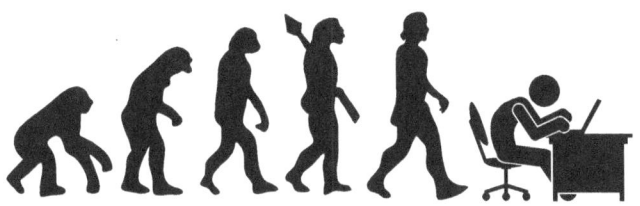

The No B.S. Guide to Becoming Human ...Again.

By Dr. Mathew Tibbitts
(Chiropractor)

Table of Contents

Before We Begin — 3
Disclaimer — 6

Part One: Core Foundations
1. Sunlight — The Forgotten Nutrient — 7
2. Earthing — Your Feet Aren't Supposed to Be in Coffins — 12
3. Water — The Liquid Foundation — 17
4. Food — You Are What You Eat (Literally) — 22

Part Two: Strength & Recovery
5. Movement & Strength — The Real Anti-Aging Secret — 27
6. Sleep & Recovery — The Forgotten Superpower — 33

Part Three: Pressure & Poisons
7. Stress — Harnessing the Pressure — 38
8. Poison — Society's Accepted Toxins = Your Declining Health — 44

Part Four: Connection & Spirit
9. Tribe & Connection — Alone We Break, Together We Thrive — 52
10. Spirit, Energy & Thoughts — Beyond the Physical — 57

Becoming Human Again — 65
Appendix: The Human Score — 66

Before We Begin

||| The State of Things

For millions of years, humans lived in rhythm with the earth. We rose with the sun, walked barefoot on the ground, hunted, gathered, ate real food, and leaned on our tribes for survival. Strength, resilience, and connection were built into daily life.

When was the last time you felt fully alive? Not just getting through the day, but strong, clear, calm, and connected? If you can't remember, you're not alone. Most people have traded health for convenience, clarity for distraction, and resilience for comfort.

I know because I see it every day. In my chiropractic clinic, people come in with chronic pain, fatigue, and anxiety. They want quick fixes, but their bodies are breaking down after years — sometimes decades — of ignoring the fundamentals of being human. I've adjusted spines, prescribed exercises, given people tools, but unless the basics are addressed — sunlight, food, sleep, movement, connection — the cycle repeats. That frustration, and my refusal to just sit by and watch it, is why I wrote this book.

||| Who the F** am I

My name is Mat. I'm 35, I live in Australia, and I'm a chiropractor. But before you picture some white-coated professional with a clipboard, let me set the record straight: I'm blunt, I swear a shit load, and I don't sugarcoat things. People either love that about me or they don't — but I've learned that honesty is what actually gets through to people.

I wasn't raised in clinics or gyms. I grew up on a small five-acre property surrounded by bushland. As a kid, I spent a lot of time outdoors— playing barefoot, helping Dad chop trees down, making adventures out of nothing. I didn't realise it at the time, but that way of living hardwired me to love nature, movement, and freedom. It gave me a sense of what it means to be human before I even knew how to put it into words.

Years later, when I became a personal trainer, I started to see just how disconnected people had become from that kind of life. For three years I watched clients push through workouts, obsess over calories, and chase body-image goals. But underneath it, most of them had no real awareness of themselves. They didn't know how to move properly, how to feel their body, or how capable they really were. I knew fitness wasn't the full answer.

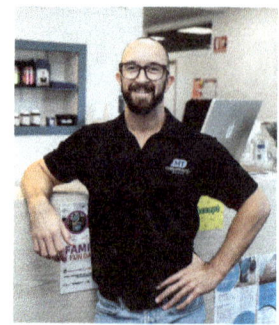

That's what led me into chiropractic. I wanted to go deeper — to really understand anatomy, physiology, neurology, and how the body works as a whole. After five years of study, I came out hungry to help people, and I still love adjusting spines and restoring movement. But here's the truth: after just four years in practice, I realised even chiropractic on its own isn't enough. I can treat the pain, but if someone goes home and keeps living disconnected from the basics — sunlight, real food, sleep, movement, connection — the same problems come straight back.

What I've learned is simple: **the body is designed to heal itself**. But we've drifted so far from what it means to be human that most people's systems barely remember how to work. That's why I wrote this book. Because I believe people are capable of so much more than just existing — and it's time we remembered how.

||| Why This Book Exists

After years of working with people — in gyms, in clinics, in conversations — I've seen the same pattern again and again: people are sick, tired, and broken down, yet they have no idea why. They think their pain or anxiety is random, or that it's just bad luck or genetics. The truth? Most of it comes from living in ways the human body was never designed to live.

Modern medicine is great at emergencies, but it's terrible at teaching people how to be human. Instead of showing us how to thrive, it offers bandaid fixes: pills for stress, orthotics for weak feet, caffeine for fatigue, surgery when everything else fails. Comfort has replaced resilience. Convenience has replaced awareness. And the result is a society that's softer, sicker, and more disconnected than ever.

That's why I wrote this book. Not to rant, and not to scare you — but to wake you up. This isn't about hacks, quick fixes, or gimmicks. It's about getting back to the fundamentals: sunlight, food, water, earth, sleep, movement, connection, spirit. The things that made us human in the first place.

This book is here because people need a no-BS guide to remember what health really is. To strip away the noise, to show you what matters, and to give you practical steps to rebuild yourself piece by piece. My goal isn't to make you perfect — it's to make you human again.

||| What You'll Get From This Book

This isn't a textbook and it's not a lecture. It's a guide. Straightforward, practical, and designed so you can read it, feel it, and actually apply it.

You'll move through each of the foundations one by one: sunlight, earthing, food, water, sleep, movement, tribe, stress, spirit, and the poisons that drag us down. In each chapter, I'll show you what's gone wrong, why it matters, and what to do about it. No fluff, just clear steps to take your health back.

And to make it real, you'll be able to measure your progress with the Human Score. It's not about perfection — it's about progress. Each point you earn is proof that you're taking back control and living more like a human again.

By the end of this book, you'll understand what your body and mind have been missing, and you'll have a plan to bring it all back. No magic pills. No quick fixes. Just the fundamentals that have always worked — the things that make you human.

||| The Choice Is Yours

Being human again is not about perfection. It's about direction. Every choice you make — what you eat, how you move, the way you rest, the way you think — nudges your body either toward health or toward breakdown. The power is in your hands, one decision at a time.

The truth is, no one is coming to save you. Your health, your clarity, your energy — they're built from your choices. Piece by piece, you can rebuild yourself. You can feel alive again. Not someday, not when it's convenient, but starting now.

This book will show you how. Not with gimmicks, but with the basics that have always worked. If you're ready to remember what it feels like to be truly human again, turn the page.

Let's get started.

||| Disclaimer

This book is for educational and informational purposes only. The content reflects general health principles and is not intended as a substitute for professional medical advice, diagnosis, or treatment. Every individual is different, and what is described in these pages may not be suitable for your personal circumstances. Before making any changes to your diet, exercise, lifestyle, or medical care, you should always consult your GP or another qualified health professional.

The references included throughout this book are provided for transparency and further reading. They do not replace professional advice or represent a complete or final authority on the subjects discussed.

While every effort has been made to ensure accuracy, neither the author nor publisher accepts any liability for injury, illness, or outcomes resulting from the application of the information presented. The responsibility for your health decisions rests with you.

Copyright © 2025 Dr. Mathew Tibbitts (Chiropractor)

All rights reserved.
No part of this book may be reproduced, distributed, or transmitted in any form or by any means — including photocopying, recording, or other electronic or mechanical methods — without the prior written permission of the author, except in the case of brief quotations used in reviews, educational purposes, or other noncommercial uses permitted by copyright law.

Published in Australia by MT Chiropractic
ABN: 56 645 006 257

This publication is for general informational purposes only and is not intended to replace professional medical advice. Always consult your qualified health practitioner or GP before making changes to your lifestyle, diet, or exercise program.

Chapter 1: Sunlight

The Forgotten Nutrient

||| The Problem

Most people today live almost entirely indoors — in dim houses, under fluorescent lights, in cars with tinted windows, faces glued to glowing screens until midnight. They treat the sun like poison, hiding from it, then wonder why they're tired, anxious, overweight, and miserable.

You're not broken. You're not cursed with "bad genes." You're just living in the dark — cut off from one of the most fundamental forces that built you. The human body is not designed for shadows. You are wired to rise with the sun, to move under its warmth, and to rest when it sets. Yet modern life has flipped that rhythm completely.

I see it every day in my clinic. People drag themselves through life, surviving on caffeine and artificial light. They wake up exhausted, work under LED glare, then stay up late scrolling under blue light that tricks their brain into thinking it's still daytime. Their body's rhythm is lost. Their hormones are confused. Their cells are starving for light.

The sun isn't your enemy — it's your oldest ally. For millions of years, it's been your compass, your clock, your natural pharmacy. Every sunrise was once a biological reset, triggering the release of hormones, regulating your sleep, your mood, and your metabolism. But now, people live as if sunlight is optional — as if they can replace it with pills, screens, and vitamin bottles. You can't. You cannot cheat nature.

The truth is simple: we've traded the rhythm of the earth for the rhythm of technology — and the cost is our vitality. We've forgotten that before there were supplements, gyms, and doctors, there was the sun. The source of all energy. The first medicine. The original life force that still powers everything living on this planet — including you.

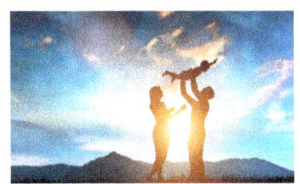

||| The Truth: Humans Are Solar Powered

For millions of years, sunlight was our fuel. It sets our body clock, drives hormone release, strengthens the immune system, and lifts our mood. Without it, our biology slips into dysfunction.

Circadian Rhythm: Morning sunlight tells your brain it's daytime. Light enters the eyes, signals the suprachiasmatic nucleus (your body's master clock), and triggers a rise in cortisol, while melatonin production shuts down [1]. That signal wakes the body, regulates energy, and sets the rhythm for every other hormone. Miss it, and your system runs out of sync all day.

Vitamin D (Hormone D): Sunlight on skin creates Vitamin D3, which functions more like a hormone than a vitamin. It regulates immune defenses, strengthens bones, and supports testosterone production [2]. Deficiency is tied to depression, fatigue, cancers, and metabolic disease [3]. Supplements can help, but they don't fully replicate what sunlight does inside your skin [4].

Mood & Brain: Sunlight also drives serotonin production, the neurotransmitter that stabilizes mood, focus, and calm. Low sunlight exposure is consistently linked to higher rates of depression and anxiety. Seasonal Affective Disorder (SAD) is a clear demonstration of what happens when the brain is starved of light [5].

In northern countries, long winter nights coincide with spikes in seasonal depression and mood disorders. In Iceland, for example, the sun may hover above the horizon for fewer than four hours on some winter days, and rates of Seasonal Affective Disorder (SAD) and mood disturbance rise significantly during these dark months — a clear reminder of how deeply humans depend on sunlight for mental and biological balance [6].

Our ancestors didn't need research papers to tell them this. They lived by the sun — rising with it, working under it, resting when it set. Their health was aligned with the cycles of light and dark.

||| The Myths That Are Costing You Your Health

"The sun causes cancer."
That's the line that's been drilled into our heads for decades — and it's only half true. Yes, chronic sunburn and reckless exposure can damage skin and increase melanoma risk. But moderate, consistent sun exposure is one of the most powerful protective forces in human biology. Research shows that people who get regular, non-burning sunlight have lower rates of several cancers, largely due to Vitamin D–related immune pathways and improved cellular repair [7]. The irony? Hiding from the sun in fear may actually increase your long-term risk of disease. The real culprits behind modern cancer and chronic illness aren't sunlight — they're processed food, alcohol, smoking, pollution, stress, and lack of movement. The sun didn't break us. Our lifestyle did.

"Sunscreen saves you."
Sunscreen has its place — but not in the way most people use it. Most commercial sunscreens block UVB rays, the very light your skin needs to create Vitamin D. Without that natural production, your immunity, hormones, and mood all take a hit. Worse still, many chemical sunscreens contain compounds like oxybenzone and octinoxate — ingredients linked to hormone disruption and environmental harm [8].

That doesn't mean you should ditch protection altogether. It means you should be smarter. Research shows sunscreen doesn't always drive Vitamin D to dangerous lows [9], but it often gives people a false sense of safety — staying out longer, burning more, and thinking they're protected. A better approach is balance: build tolerance gradually, seek shade during peak UV hours, wear protective clothing, and if needed, use mineral-based sunscreens made from zinc oxide or titanium dioxide. Let your skin see the sun — just not to the point of damage.

"Sunglasses are harmless."
Your eyes are more than lenses — they're light sensors that regulate your entire biology. When sunlight reaches the retina, it signals your brain to adjust hormones like cortisol, melatonin, serotonin — and even melanocyte-stimulating hormones that help your skin prepare for UV exposure [10]. Block that light all day with sunglasses, and your body never receives the full "daytime signal." Your brain thinks it's darker than it is, and your skin may not activate its natural defense mechanisms as effectively. You might look cool, but your biology gets confused. Wear sunglasses when the glare is harsh or when driving, but not as a reflex every time you step outside. Morning and late-afternoon light, in particular, should reach your eyes directly (without staring into the sun) — it's one of the simplest, most powerful ways to reset your system and feel alive again.

We've been taught to fear the sun, to hide from the very thing that keeps us alive. But sunlight isn't the problem — our disconnection from it is. We've traded natural light for artificial glow and wonder why we feel drained. Reconnecting with the sun isn't about chasing a tan — it's about remembering what it means to be human.

||| The Fix: How to Reclaim the Sun

- **Morning Sun (10–20 minutes):** Get outside within 30 minutes of waking. No sunglasses. Let the light hit your eyes and skin. This anchors your circadian rhythm and sets your hormones for the day.
- **Skin in the Game:** Expose as much skin as you reasonably can — arms, legs, torso. The more surface area, the more Vitamin D your body can generate.
- **Midday Boost (10–15 minutes):** Around solar noon, UVB is strongest and Vitamin D production peaks. Just a short exposure here can produce thousands of IU of Vitamin D.
- **Build Tolerance:** If you've avoided the sun for years, start with 5–10 minutes and build gradually. Burn = damage. Tan = resilience.
- **Skip the Chemicals:** Use natural protection like hats or clothes if you're outside for long periods. Reserve sunscreen for special situations, and choose zinc oxide–based formulas instead of chemical cocktails.

||| The Plan: Add It to Your Human Score

1. **Morning Sunlight:** Get at least 10 minutes of natural sunlight on your skin and eyes within 30 minutes of waking. No sunglasses. *(1 point)*
2. **Midday Exposure:** Expose as much skin as possible to the midday sun for 10–20 minutes, depending on your skin type and tolerance. *(1 point)*
3. **Minimal Sunglasses Use:** Only wear sunglasses when glare is unbearable. Let your eyes take in natural light to keep your circadian rhythm sharp. *(1 point)*

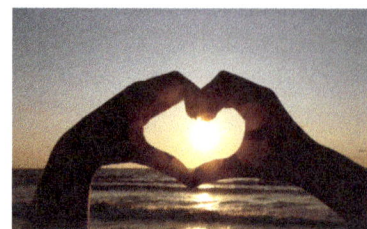

||| Final Word

The sun has never stopped rising — we just stopped showing up for it.

We traded the fire in the sky for fluorescent bulbs and phone screens, for alarms that rip us out of sleep instead of light that gently wakes us. We forgot what it feels like to be charged by the world around us — to stand barefoot in the morning, breathing the same air our ancestors did, while the first rays of light remind every cell that we're still alive.

You don't need another caffeine hit or a supplement to feel human again. You need the source. The same energy that fuels forests, oceans, and life itself is waiting outside your door every morning, asking nothing from you but to show up.

When sunlight touches your skin, your body remembers. Your hormones align. Your brain clears. Your spirit wakes. That's not magic — that's nature doing what it's always done.

So start tomorrow. Step outside. Feel the warmth on your face and let it remind you of what you are — not a machine built to grind, but a human built to live.

Because before you were tired, busy, or lost —you were sunlight, turned into life.

And it's time to remember that again.

||| References

1. Patton & Hastings. The suprachiasmatic nucleus: master regulators of circadian clock in mammals. Current Biology.
2. Holick MF. Sunlight, Vitamin D and Human Health. Nutrients.
3. Garland CF et al. Vitamin D and prevention of cancer: global perspective. American Journal of Public Health.
4. John EM et al. Sunlight and mortality: epidemiological evidence.
5. Lam RW, Levitt AJ. Canadian consensus guidelines for the treatment of Seasonal Affective Disorder.
6. Magnússon A, Axelsson J, Karlsson MM, Örnolfsdóttir H. Prevalence of seasonal affective disorder in Iceland. Journal of Affective Disorders. 2000;58(3):235–245.
7. Mohr SB et al. Is prevention of cancer by sun exposure more than just the effect of vitamin D?
8. Krause M et al. Sunscreens: are they endocrine disruptors?
9. Young AR et al. Sunscreens and Vitamin D status. British Journal of Dermatology.
10. Innate Fertility. Are your sunglasses making your sunburn worse? 2023.

Chapter 2: 🌍 Earthing

Your Feet Aren't Supposed to Be in Coffins

||| The Problem

No other species avoids the ground beneath it like we do. Every animal walks, crawls, runs, or rests in direct contact with the Earth. Humans? We've chosen to insulate ourselves from it. Rubber soles, concrete, carpet, asphalt — all these layers cut us off from the very surface our bodies were designed to connect with. Step by step, we've broken a relationship that kept us strong for millions of years.

In the clinic, I see the price of that disconnection. People come in with stubborn back pain, grinding hips, chronic fatigue, and anxiety. I can adjust their spines, mobilize their joints, prescribe exercises — but none of it sticks if the foundation is wrong. Weak, disconnected feet send a chain reaction of dysfunction up through the body. The skeleton compensates, the nervous system stays on edge, and people wonder why they never feel truly "fixed."

Look around in any shopping centre, gym, or office. You'll spot collapsed arches, twisted toes, knees buckling inward, hips tilting forward, shoulders slumping. Entire postures breaking down in slow motion. It's not just cosmetic — it's structural failure. And at the root of it? Feet that have been trapped in stiff, cushioned shoes for decades, cut off from the Earth they were meant to grip and draw strength from.

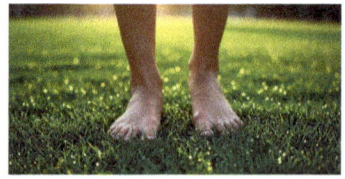

||| The Truth: Humans Are Wired to the Earth

We like to think we're "modern" and "advanced," but the human body hasn't changed in 200,000 years. It's still the same biology, running on the same laws of physics. And physics says this: the Earth is electric.

The Earth carries a natural negative charge. When your bare skin touches the ground — grass, dirt, sand — electrons move into your body. This isn't mystical. It's measurable. These electrons act like nature's antioxidants, neutralising free radicals before they can damage your tissues [1]. Chronic inflammation — the root of pain, arthritis, heart disease, even cancer — is fuelled by free radicals. Touching the Earth literally gives your body the electrical balance it needs to calm that fire.

Inflammation and Circulation: Research backs this up. A 2013 study led by Dr. Gaétan Chevalier found that grounding significantly reduced blood viscosity — meaning the blood became thinner and flowed more easily [2]. Sticky blood clogs vessels, raises blood pressure, and starves tissues of oxygen. Smooth, free-flowing blood delivers oxygen and nutrients efficiently, keeping joints supple, muscles energised, and the heart under less strain.

Pain and Sleep: Another study published in 2004 (Ober, Chevalier, & Zucker) showed that people who slept on grounding mats had reduced cortisol levels at night and reported better sleep [3]. Chronic pain isn't just about tissue damage — it's about your nervous system being stuck in a loop of over-sensitivity. Grounding helps regulate cortisol, the body's main stress hormone. Resetting this cycle allows people to fall asleep faster, stay asleep longer, and wake up more refreshed.

Nervous System Balance: Your body runs on two gears: fight-or-flight (sympathetic) and rest-and-digest (parasympathetic). Modern life keeps most people stuck in the first gear — tense, reactive, anxious. Grounding has been shown to tip the balance back, calming the sympathetic drive and activating parasympathetic recovery. A 2010 pilot study found measurable changes in heart rate variability (a key marker of nervous system balance) after just 40 minutes of earthing [4]. That deep breath you feel when you kick your shoes off in the grass isn't in your head — it's your biology recalibrating to the Earth's field.

And honestly? You don't need a scientific journal to prove it to yourself. Think of the last time you stood barefoot on cool grass at sunrise, sank your toes into beach sand, or walked across damp earth after rain. That deep exhale, that calm spreading through your chest — that's your nervous system remembering what connection feels like. You weren't designed to be cut off. You were designed to be plugged in.

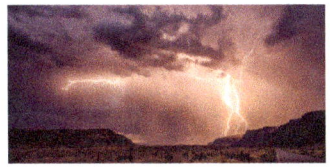

||| Shoes — Coffins for Your Feet

Your feet are engineering masterpieces: 26 bones, 33 joints, over 100 muscles, tendons, and ligaments. They are designed for movement, shock absorption, balance, and feedback. They're meant to mold to uneven ground, grip surfaces, and communicate with your brain to adjust posture.

But what do we do? We stuff them in stiff, narrow, cushioned coffins.

- **Narrow Toe Boxes:** Squeeze your toes together, and you rob them of their natural spread. That spread stabilizes your gait. Without it, balance suffers, arches collapse, bunions form, and the dysfunction ripples upward into knees, hips, and spine.
- **Elevated Heels:** Even a "small" heel lift in casual sneakers tips your pelvis forward, shortens your calves, and locks your lower back into extension [5].
- **Over-Cushioning:** Cushion feels good short-term, but long-term it weakens the feet. Just like a hand kept in a cast will waste away, feet stuck in padding lose their strength.

A 2010 study comparing barefoot vs. shoe-wearing populations found something fascinating: people who grew up barefoot had strong, wide, resilient feet — no bunions, no collapsed arches. Shoe-wearing populations? Widespread deformities and weaknesses [6].

And then there are orthotics. They're handed out like candy in clinics, as if sliding a piece of plastic into your shoe will magically fix years of dysfunction. But orthotics don't rebuild your feet — they babysit them. They can help elderly patients or those with severe deformities, but for most people, they just reinforce weakness [7]. Over time, the muscles waste away, the tendons stiffen, and the dependency grows. Orthotics don't give you freedom — they lock you into reliance.

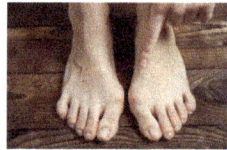

||| The Fix: How to Reconnect and Rebuild

- **Daily Barefoot Time:** Start with 10 minutes barefoot on natural ground each day. Grass, dirt, sand, soil — not concrete. Let your nervous system recalibrate.
- **Flat Shoes:** Look for shoes with wide toe boxes, zero drop (flat sole), and flexible bottoms. Brands like VivoBarefoot, Xero, or Lems let your feet function as intended.
- **Strengthen the Feet:** Try toe spacers, calf raises, towel scrunches, tip-toe walking, and barefoot balancing. Orthotics are not the long-term answer for most people — strength is.
- **Reduce Cushion:** Gradually reduce time in over-cushioned runners or "supportive" shoes. The goal isn't support — it's strength.
- **Earthing Mats:** If you can't get outside daily, grounding mats provide a substitute. Research shows they can lower cortisol, improve sleep, and reduce inflammation [8].

||| The Plan: Add It to Your Human Score

1. **Daily Barefoot Time:** Spend at least 10 minutes with bare skin touching natural ground (grass, dirt, sand, soil). *(1 point)*
2. **Flat Shoes, Not Heels:** Wear flat-soled shoes (zero or minimal heel lift) throughout the day. Minimalist shoes are ideal, but the main rule is no elevated heels. *(1 point)*
3. **Strengthen the Feet:** Do one drill to build foot strength and alignment — tip-toe walking, toe spacers, towel scrunches, or barefoot balance work. *(1 point)*

||| Final Word

Your feet aren't supposed to be weak stubs stuffed into fashion coffins. They're meant to be powerful, resilient, and connected. Right now, most people's feet look more like broken tools than strong, natural foundations. And when the foundation is broken, the whole house is unstable.

Orthotics, painkillers, and surgeries won't save you. They're patches on a sinking ship. What you need is to reclaim what's yours — strong, adaptable feet that connect you to the Earth itself.

Tomorrow, take your shoes off. Step onto the earth. Feel it. At first it might feel awkward, even vulnerable — but that's the point. You're reconnecting with something bigger than you, something your body has been craving for decades.

This isn't nostalgia. It's biology. You're not designed for rubber soles and concrete floors. You're designed for Earth, balance, strength. Reconnect with it, and you'll feel the shift through your entire body.

Wake up your feet, and you'll wake up yourself.

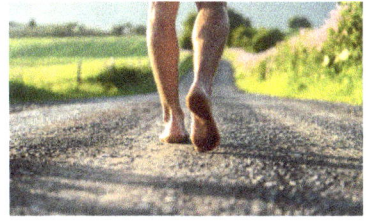

||| References

1. Oschman JL. Perspective: Energy medicine, the scientific basis of earthing. Journal of Alternative and Complementary Medicine.
2. Chevalier G, et al. Earthing (Grounding) the Human Body Reduces Blood Viscosity—a Major Factor in Cardiovascular Disease. J Altern Complement Med. 2013.
3. Ober C, Chevalier G, Zucker M. Grounding the human body during sleep reduces night-time cortisol levels and improves sleep, pain, and stress. J Altern Complement Med. 2004.
4. Chevalier G. The effects of earthing on human physiology. Subtle Energies & Energy Medicine. 2010.
5. Nigg BM, et al. Footwear and postural alignment: biomechanical consequences of elevated heels. Gait & Posture.
6. Rao UB, Joseph B. The influence of footwear on the prevalence of flat foot: a survey of 2300 children. J Bone Joint Surg Br. 1992.
7. Richards CE, Magin PJ, Callister R. Is orthotic therapy effective in treating lower limb conditions? A systematic review. Br J Sports Med.
8. Chevalier G, Sinatra ST, Oschman JL, Delany RM. Earthing: Health implications of reconnecting the human body to the Earth's surface electrons. J Environ Public Health. 2012.

Chapter 3: 💧 Water

The Liquid Foundation

||| The Problem

Most people think water is just water — turn on the tap, fill a glass, and you're set. But what comes out of modern taps is a far cry from the quality spring water humans have evolved with. Instead of mineral-rich, living water, we're drinking a chemical brew that fills the stomach but starves the cells.

Our ancestors drank from springs, rivers, and streams. Living water — mineral-rich, flowing, filtered naturally through rock and earth. Today we drink chemical cocktails pumped through old pipes, laced with chlorine, fluoride, pesticides, heavy metals, and god knows what else [1]. It's water that fills the glass but barely nourishes the body.

Dehydration is more common than most people think. Even mild dehydration — as little as 1–2% loss of body weight in water — reduces mental clarity, slows reaction times, and increases fatigue [2]. At 3–4%, performance drops, headaches strike, mood crashes, and digestion stalls [3]. Chronic low-grade dehydration is linked to joint pain, poor fascia mobility, kidney stress, and constipation [4]. And here's the truth most people miss: your body can't heal properly if it's dehydrated. Water is the medium for every repair process in your system — starve it, and you cripple your own recovery.

The flip side? Proper hydration is one of the fastest ways to feel better. Balanced hydration improves joint lubrication, spinal disc health, blood flow, temperature regulation, and even neurotransmitter function in the brain [5]. A hydrated body is an energetic body — but only if the water you're drinking actually nourishes your cells.

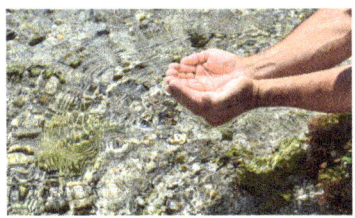

||| The Truth: Tap Water Isn't Just "Water"

Let's break it down:

- **Chlorine:** Added to kill bacteria. It also kills beneficial gut bacteria when consumed regularly, and long-term exposure is linked to higher risks of certain cancers [6].
- **Fluoride:** Promoted for "dental health," but studies link overexposure to thyroid dysfunction, lowered IQ in children, and bone issues [7]. Australia and the USA are two of the most fluoridated-water nations in the world.
- **Heavy Metals:** Old pipes leach lead, copper, and other metals into the supply. Chronic low-level exposure contributes to neurological issues and developmental delays [8].
- **Pesticides & Chemicals:** Agricultural runoff ends up in reservoirs. Traces of herbicides, pharmaceuticals, and industrial waste are routinely found in municipal water supplies [9].

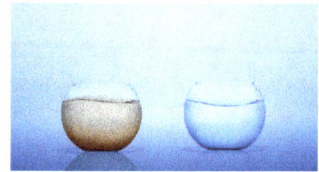

That's not hydration — that's low-dose poisoning.

And then there's bottled water. Tests have shown microplastics in over 90% of samples worldwide [10]. Heating plastic bottles in cars or shipping containers makes it worse. You end up drinking plastic fibers and endocrine-disrupting chemicals along with your "pure" water.

And this idea that we all need to chug three litres of water every day? That's not natural. Our ancestors weren't walking around with water bottles strapped to their hips. They drank when they were thirsty — and their water actually hydrated them.

Modern water is so depleted, so filtered, so chemically altered, that it doesn't hold the minerals our bodies need. Electrolytes — sodium, potassium, magnesium, calcium — are stripped away. That's why you can drink liters of tap water and still feel thirsty, still get cramps, still feel flat [11].

||| The Science: Do You Really Need 3 Litres a Day?

The "8 glasses a day" or "3 litres a day" rule is a myth. Studies show daily hydration needs depend on diet, activity, and environment — not some arbitrary number [12]. If you eat fresh fruit and vegetables (which are water-rich), your body actually needs less drinking water.

So why do people today feel like they need gallons? Because modern water is empty. It lacks minerals, and it's full of contaminants that force the kidneys to work harder. Your body screams for more, but it's not real hydration — it's your system trying to flush the junk.

Research from the National Academies of Sciences (2004) shows that total hydration needs vary widely depending on diet, activity, and climate — and much of it comes from food [13]. Fresh fruit, vegetables, and even meat contribute water. Ancient humans who ate whole foods didn't need to carry a drink bottle all day.

Modern humans need more water partly because our diets are dry (processed food contains little water) and partly because the water itself is empty. Without minerals, water moves through the body faster, leading to constant thirst and diluted electrolytes [14]. That's why electrolytes matter — they don't just "add flavour." They help water stay in your cells, where it actually counts.

||| Signs of Hydration: How to Know if You're Actually Watered

Most people don't know how to read their own hydration. They either chug litres mindlessly or barely drink at all. But your body gives clear signals if you pay attention.

- **Urine Colour:**
    - Pale Yellow = healthy hydration.
    - Clear = looks good, but usually means you're flushing water straight through without absorbing it (often due to low minerals) [15].
    - Dark Yellow/Amber = dehydration. Your body is conserving water because there isn't enough coming in.
- **Skin & Hair:** Dry or flaky skin, itchy scalp, or beard dandruff can all signal low hydration. Hydrated skin is supple and resilient [16].
- **Lips & Mouth:** Constantly dry lips or sticky mouth = your body is prioritizing water for survival functions, not comfort.
- **Energy & Focus:** Even mild dehydration (1–2% body weight loss) impacts brain function and mood [17].

Tracking these signs daily is far more useful than following "8 glasses a day." Hydration isn't about how much you drink — it's about how much your body absorbs.

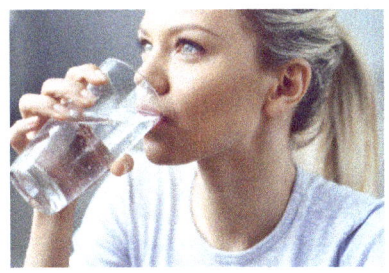

||| The Fix: How to Drink Like a Human

- **Filter Your Water:** Even cheap filters (like Brita or ceramic units) reduce chlorine, heavy metals, and microplastics. A reverse-osmosis system or high-quality carbon filter is ideal.
- **Upgrade With Minerals:** Add electrolytes daily. This isn't just for athletes — it's for anyone living on depleted modern water and food. Use clean electrolyte powders or add a pinch of sea salt and a squeeze of lemon.
- **Ditch Plastic Bottles:** Use stainless steel or glass bottles. If you must buy bottled water, choose brands that use glass or BPA-free bottles, and don't store them in heat.
- **Spring Water Where Possible:** If you can access a spring or mountain source, this is the gold standard. Mineral-rich, structured, living water.
- **Drink With Purpose:** Stop mindlessly chugging. Drink when thirsty, support hydration with electrolytes, and get water through food (fruits, vegetables, soups).

||| The Plan: Add It to Your Human Score

1. **Filtered Water (all day):** Ditch the tap water and drink filtered water throughout the day. Every sip supports your cells instead of drowning them in chemicals. *(1 point)*
2. **Electrolyte Support (once daily):** Add a pinch of natural sea salt/celtic salt, trace minerals, or electrolytes once a day to restore what sweat, stress, and caffeine drain from your system. *(1 point)*
3. **Plastic-Free (glass/steel only):** Switch to glass or stainless steel for both storage and drinking. It's a small shift that keeps your water — and your body — clean. *(1 point)*

||| Final Word

Water is life. It makes up your cells, your blood, your brain. It carries oxygen, clears waste, drives energy. But modern humans are guzzling poisoned, depleted versions of it — and calling that hydration.

It doesn't have to be complicated. Filter your water. Add minerals back in. Respect it as the life source it is.

Because here's the blunt truth: you're not tired because you need more coffee. You're tired because your cells are dehydrated with garbage water.

Fix your water, and everything else in your body works better. Energy lifts. Joints loosen. Focus sharpens. Digestion smooths. Every cell thanks you.

Humans are 70% water. If your water is poor, your health will be too. But if your water is strong, so are you.

||| References

1. Whelton AJ, et al. Water quality issues in distribution systems: corrosion, contamination, and health risks. Water Res.
2. Grandjean AC, Grandjean NR. Dehydration and cognitive performance. J Am Coll Nutr. 2007.
3. Shirreffs SM, Sawka MN. Fluid and electrolyte needs for training, competition, and recovery. J Sports Sci. 2011.
4. Popkin BM, et al. Water, hydration, and health. Nutr Rev. 2010.
5. Armstrong LE. Hydration assessment techniques. Nutr Rev. 2005.
6. Villanueva CM, et al. Bladder cancer and exposure to water disinfection by-products through ingestion, bathing, showering, and swimming in pools. Am J Epidemiol. 2007.
7. Peckham S, Awofeso N. Water fluoridation: a critical review of the physiological effects of ingested fluoride. Sci World J. 2014.
8. Bellinger DC. Neurological and behavioral consequences of childhood lead exposure. PLoS Med. 2008.
9. Benotti MJ, et al. Pharmaceuticals and endocrine disrupting compounds in US drinking water. Environ Sci Technol. 2009.
10. Mason SA, et al. Synthetic polymer contamination in bottled water. Front Chem. 2018.
11. Costill DL, et al. Effects of repeated days of intensified training on muscle glycogen and performance. Med Sci Sports Exerc. 1988.
12. EFSA Panel on Dietetic Products. Scientific Opinion on Dietary Reference Values for water. EFSA Journal. 2010.
13. National Academies of Sciences. Dietary Reference Intakes for Water, Potassium, Sodium, Chloride, and Sulfate. 2004.
14. Jequier E, Constant F. Water as an essential nutrient: the physiological basis of hydration. Eur J Clin Nutr. 2010.
15. Armstrong LE, et al. Urinary indices of hydration status. Int J Sport Nutr. 1994.
16. Proksch E, et al. The skin: an indispensable barrier. Exp Dermatol. 2008.
17. Masento NA, et al. Effects of hydration status on cognitive performance and mood. Br J Nutr. 2014.

Chapter 4: 🍽 Food

You Are What You Eat, Literally.

||| The Problem

Food is the most important material of life. Without food, we die. Every cell in your body, every thought in your mind, every movement you make is built from what you put in your mouth. Yet somehow, in the modern world, food has been downgraded to an afterthought — an inconvenience squeezed between meetings, work shifts, and commutes.

People spend more time researching a new phone than they do questioning what fuels their body. They grab takeout on the way home, scroll while eating, and wash it down with soda or beer. Then they wonder why they feel like garbage.

Here's the blunt truth: you are what you eat — literally. Your blood, your bones, your brain, even your DNA is made from the nutrients (or lack of them) that you consume. If you eat shit, you build a shit body and a shit mind. It's that simple.

And yet, the modern world has made eating well harder than ever. Supermarkets are full of processed "food-like products" engineered for taste and shelf life, not nourishment. We eat strawberries in winter shipped halfway across the planet, instead of seasonal food that syncs with our biology. We've forgotten the simplicity of our ancestors: if it didn't grow in the ground, fall from a tree, or walk on four legs, it wasn't food.

We've traded the most essential part of human life — food — for convenience. And the cost is showing up in our bodies and minds more than ever.

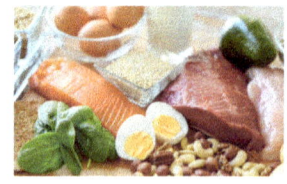

||| The Truth: What Food Really Is

Humans evolved eating what nature provided: meat, fruit, vegetables. Real food, in its natural form. Our genes, our microbiome, and our metabolism are still wired for this. But instead of aligning with that design, modern diets now revolve around ultra-processed grains, industrial seed oils, refined sugar, and chemical additives — a mismatch that drives metabolic disease, obesity, and chronic inflammation [1,2].

Look around in a shopping centre and you'll see the result. Bloated guts, skinny arms, weak postures, tired eyes. For millions of years, men were strong to hunt and protect, women were active, calm, and nurturing. Now, both sexes slump through life looking half-human. Evolution's proud arc — from ape to man — seems to have taken a detour into hunched, inflamed, robotic weakness.

||| The Gut–Brain Connection: Feeding Your Mind

Most people think food is only about their waistline or energy levels. But here's the truth: what you eat literally builds your brain. The gut and the brain are hard-wired together by the vagus nerve and by chemical messengers made in the gut microbiome [3,4]. About 90% of the body's serotonin is produced in the gut by enterochromaffin cells influenced by microbes — which helps explain why gut health shows up as mood, focus, and calm (or the lack of it) [5].

When your gut is inflamed, when your microbiome is out of balance, when your food quality is poor — your brain pays the price. Brain fog, mood swings, anxiety, depression — they don't just "happen." They're often fuelled by what's happening in your digestive system [4,6].

Research is piling up showing that diet and gut dysfunction are linked to conditions such as:

- **ADHD and autism spectrum disorders:** Altered gut microbiomes are frequently observed, and dietary/probiotic interventions can influence symptoms in some people (diet isn't "the cause," but the gut–brain axis shapes how these conditions present) [7,8].
- **Depression and anxiety:** Systemic inflammation and microbiome imbalance disrupt serotonin pathways and stress signaling [6,9].
- **Alzheimer's and dementia:** Chronic inflammation and insulin resistance from poor diets are major drivers of neurodegeneration; Alzheimer's is increasingly discussed as "type 3 diabetes" in the literature [10,11].

Think about that: the way you eat today doesn't just affect your body; it lays the foundation for how your mind will work tomorrow — and decades from now.

Your brain is not separate from your stomach. Feed your gut garbage, and your brain will process garbage. Feed your gut nutrients, and your brain will have the raw materials it needs to build memory, focus, mood, and resilience.

||| Resetting the Gut

Food isn't just fuel. It's also how your body communicates with itself. The gut isn't a simple tube — it's a living ecosystem of bacteria, fungi, and cells that directly influence brain, mood, and immunity [3,4].

When you eat poorly — processed foods, alcohol, artificial additives — you don't just miss out on nutrients. You disrupt the microbiome. Bad actors take over, the gut lining becomes leaky and inflamed, and nutrient absorption tanks. Sometimes the system needs a reset — like clearing weeds before planting again.

Ways to initiate a reset:
- **Fasting:** Strategic breaks from eating (intermittent, 24-hour, or longer under professional supervision) can improve insulin sensitivity, calm inflammation, and allow gut lining repair [12].
- **Short cleanses/elimination phases:** Removing processed foods, sugar, alcohol, and stimulants while focusing on simple, whole foods can rapidly improve energy, digestion, and mental clarity [13].
- **Colonics:** A direct way to flush the colon. Some people report symptomatic relief and mental clarity. Evidence is limited and it's not for everyone — medical guidance is advised, especially if you have GI conditions [14].

Think of it like gardening: don't dump fertiliser onto poisoned, compacted soil. Turn it over, clear the weeds, reset the environment — then add nutrients. That's when the system thrives.

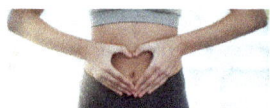

||| The Cost of Disconnecting From Real Food

When you cut corners with food, your body pays the price. Poor digestion, poor absorption, and a starving microbiome mean your cells aren't getting the raw materials they need. That shows up everywhere:

- **Weak bones and muscles** from mineral and protein deficits.
- **Fatigue and brain fog** from unstable blood sugar and chronic inflammation [2].
- **Hormonal chaos** when amino acids, fats, and micronutrients are inadequate for hormone synthesis.
- **Higher disease risk** from ultra-processed diets increasing energy intake and weight gain, pushing metabolic disease [1].

And let's not forget: poisons like alcohol and smoking add fuel to the fire — they deplete nutrients, inflame tissues, and trash digestion [15,16]. You can't expect your food to nourish you if you're constantly poisoning the system.

||| The Fix: How to Reclaim Food as Fuel

- **Eat Real Food:** If it didn't come from the ground, a tree, or an animal in its natural form, it's not food. Meat, fruit, vegetables — simple as that.
- **Eat Seasonal:** Choose food grown in rhythm with the earth. Seasonal eating aligns nutrient profiles and supports metabolic rhythms [17].
- **Cook, Don't Just Consume:** Preparing food re-establishes your relationship with it. Slow down. Smell, touch, taste. The process matters.
- **Hydrate With Purpose:** Water supports digestion and absorption. Soda, alcohol, and energy drinks destroy it [15].
- **Respect the Environment of Eating:** No shoveling food while scrolling. Sit, chew, breathe, connect. Your state while eating affects digestion via the nervous system [3].
- **Reset the Gut:** Fasting, short cleanses, or (with guidance) colonics can give your gut the reset it needs so new nutrients land in healthy soil [12–14].
- **Ditch the Processed Crap:** Real food doesn't need a label. If it comes in a box, has a barcode, or lists ingredients you can't pronounce, it's not food — it's chemistry [1].

||| The Plan: Add It to Your Human Score

1. **Eat Real Food (meat, fruit, vegetables):** Every meal today comes from nature. If it grew in the ground, fell from a tree, or walked the earth, it counts. (1 point)
2. **Zero Processed Foods:** No bread, no soft drinks, no packaged "food-like" products. If it came with a barcode or a long list of ingredients, skip it. (1 point)
3. **Conscious Eating:** Sit down, slow down, and treat eating as a ritual. No scrolling, no TV, no distractions — just you, your food, and the purpose of fueling your body. (1 point)

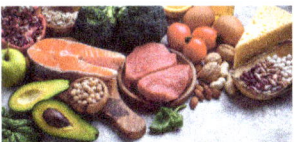

||| The Final Word

Food isn't complicated. It's not about calorie spreadsheets, fad diets, or the latest supplement hack. It's about giving your body and brain the raw materials they need to thrive.

The modern world makes it easy to forget, but deep down you already know what food is. Real food grows, moves, and nourishes. Fake food comes in boxes and barcodes.

You have a choice every time you sit down to eat: to build health or to build disease. To sharpen your mind or to fog it. To strengthen your future or to weaken it.

Your body will become what you feed it. Your brain will think with the fuel you provide. If you want clarity, resilience, and vitality — start with the food on your plate.

||| References

1. Hall KD, et al. Ultra-processed diets cause excess calorie intake and weight gain. Cell Metab. 2019.
2. Ludwig DS, Ebbeling CB. The carbohydrate-insulin model: a physiological perspective on obesity. JAMA Intern Med. 2018.
3. Mayer EA. The neurobiology of the gut–brain axis. Nat Rev Gastroenterol Hepatol. 2011.
4. Cryan JF, Dinan TG. Mind-altering microorganisms: the impact of the gut microbiota on brain and behaviour. Nat Rev Neurosci. 2012; and Cryan JF et al., 2019 update.
5. Gershon MD, Tack J. The serotonin signaling system: enteric sources and functions. Gastroenterology. 2007; Yano JM et al. 2015 (microbiota regulate gut 5-HT).
6. Foster JA, Neufeld K-AM. Gut–brain axis: how the microbiome influences anxiety and depression. Trends Neurosci. 2013.
7. Vuong HE, Hsiao EY. Emerging roles for the gut microbiome in autism spectrum disorder. Dev Disabil Res Rev. / Sci Transl Med. 2017.
8. Bundgaard-Nielsen C, et al. Gut microbiota profiles in ADHD. Sci Rep. 2020.
9. Dantzer R, et al. From inflammation to sickness and depression. Nat Rev Neurosci. 2008.

Chapter 5: Movement & Strength

The Real Anit-Aging Secret

||| The Problem

Humans were designed to move, but modern life has turned us into statues. We sit in cars, we sit at desks, we sit on couches, we sit at dinner tables. The average person spends more hours parked on their arse than they do walking, lifting, carrying, or playing.

And here's the problem: the less you move, the weaker you get. The weaker you get, the more your joints, ligaments, and bones take the load. That's when the body starts to break down — arthritis, disc problems, tendon issues, pain that never leaves. People think they're "just getting old," but most of the time they're just weak [1].

What society doesn't realise is that work is physical activity, no matter what job you do. Even if you sit all day, your muscles are constantly firing to hold you upright against gravity. They never switch off. They get tired, they get sore, they get overloaded.

So the real question is this: is your body strong enough for your job? For most people, the answer is no. Whether it's a tradie on the tools, a nurse on the ward, or an office worker at a desk, the body is under load all day long. If your muscles aren't strong enough to carry it, the strain goes somewhere else — into your joints, your discs, your fascia. That's when the breakdown begins.

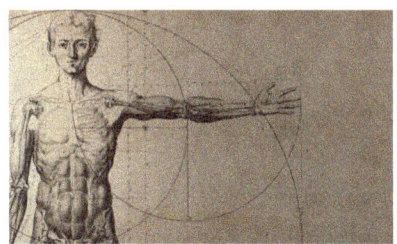

||| The Truth: Strength is Survival

Your muscles aren't just decoration — they're your body's scaffolding. They hold your skeleton upright, stabilise your joints, and absorb the forces of gravity and life. Without strong muscles, every movement you make — standing, bending, carrying groceries — dumps load into your joints, discs, and ligaments. These structures weren't designed to take that punishment. That's why weak bodies degenerate faster [2].

But muscles do more than just protect. Movement is what keeps your blood and lymph flowing. Your heart pumps blood, but it relies on muscular contractions to squeeze vessels and push circulation out to every corner of the body. And your lymphatic system — the network that clears waste and supports immunity — doesn't even have a pump. It only moves when you move [3]. That means if you sit still all day, your waste products stagnate, your immune defence slows, and your tissues literally drown in their own rubbish.

Then there's fascia — the connective web that links every muscle, bone, and organ together. It's like a wrapping of plastic wrap; but it's alive, full of nerves and fluid. When you move often and in varied ways, fascia stays hydrated and pliable. When you sit still or repeat the same motions over and over, it stiffens and sticks, strangling your mobility [4]. That's why varied, loaded, dynamic movement isn't optional — it's essential for staying pain-free and functional.

And here's the truth: your muscles are always switched on. Even at rest, they're holding you upright against gravity. That means if your muscles are weak, they fatigue faster, and the load that is put through them starts to distribute into the bone, joints and ligaments.

||| Pain: The Body's Alarm System

Pain isn't random. It's your body's defence mechanism, a built-in alarm telling you something isn't right. Yet modern society treats pain like a mistake — something to medicate away, silence, or ignore. Pop a pill, keep grinding, hope it disappears. But pain doesn't show up without reason.

Most chronic pain isn't caused by some "mystery condition." It comes from weakness, poor mechanics, or overload. When your muscles can't handle the demand of your job or lifestyle, the strain shifts into ligaments, joints, and discs. That's when the alarms go off. Low back pain, neck stiffness, shoulder aches — they're the body's way of saying, "I can't keep this up" [5].

Pain is feedback. It's not the enemy, it's the message. Treating pain with pills without addressing the cause is like smashing the smoke alarm while the house burns down. The problem doesn't go away — it gets worse.

When you build strength, restore balance, and move the way your body was designed to, the nervous system relaxes. The body feels safe again. And often, the pain signal fades — not because it was "masked," but because the alarm is no longer needed.

||| The Cost of Weakness & The Power of Strength

Weakness doesn't just make you feel tired — it accelerates your breakdown. If your muscles can't carry the load, your joints, discs, and ligaments are forced to. And those tissues aren't designed for constant impact. Over time, they fray, thin, and collapse under the pressure.

- **Degeneration:** Arthritis, disc herniations, bone spurs — these aren't random curses of "old age." They're the end result of years of weak muscles dumping load into passive structures. Strong muscles protect; weak muscles destroy [2].
- **Repetitive Strain:** Tradesmen wear out their shoulders, backs, and knees. Office workers wreck their necks, wrists, and hips. Repetition without balance is the perfect recipe for pain.
- **Falls & Independence:** Weak legs are the number one predictor of falls in older age. And the statistics are brutal: a fall that breaks a hip often marks the beginning of the end. Strength literally decides whether you'll live independently or rely on others [6].
- **Circulation & Recovery:** Without muscular contraction, blood and lymph flow stagnate. Healing slows. Waste builds up. Inflammation lingers.
- **Use It or Lose It:** The body doesn't store strength for later. If you don't use it, you lose it. Muscle mass, fascia elasticity, bone density, coordination — all fade unless you stress them regularly [7].

But here's the other side of the story — the part most people overlook: Strength and movement go beyond the physical frame — it shapes every system in the body, from metabolism to immunity.

- **Metabolic Power:** Muscle tissue is a metabolic engine. The more you have, the more efficiently your body handles glucose, the more insulin-sensitive you are, and the lower your risk of type 2 diabetes [8].
- **Bone Density:** Bones don't stay strong on their own. They respond to stress. Resistance training signals them to thicken, harden, and reinforce. That's why strength training is the number one protection against osteoporosis [9].
- **Hormonal Health:** Movement improves testosterone, growth hormone, and estrogen balance. These aren't just "sex hormones" — they're key drivers of energy, mood, recovery, and resilience [10].
- **Longevity:** Studies show that grip strength, leg strength, and muscle mass are some of the strongest predictors of how long and how well people live [11]. Strong people live longer, period.
- **Quality of Life:** Beyond the science, strength makes life easier. Carrying groceries, climbing stairs, playing with kids — all of it feels lighter when your body is strong.

I see both sides of this coin every day in clinic. Weak patients break down early, suffering from pain, degeneration, and loss of independence. Stronger patients recover faster, resist injury, and stay active well into older age. Weakness is a slow decline. Strength is a buffer against time.

||| The Fix: Move Like a Human

The good news? Strength isn't lost forever. The body is ridiculously adaptable. No matter your age, no matter your job, no matter how long you've been weak — if you stress the body the right way, it responds. Muscle grows. Fascia loosens. Joints feel safer. Pain signals calm down.

But you don't need a fancy program or some influencer's "secret." You need the basics — the movements humans have always done.

- **Lift Heavy (For You):** Resistance training isn't optional. Your muscles need load to stay alive. That might be barbells in a gym, bodyweight at home, resistance bands, kettlebells, or even lifting logs and rocks in the backyard. The tool doesn't matter — the principle does. Stress the muscles, and they adapt.
- **Move in All Planes:** Life isn't straight lines. Yet most people only sit, stand, or walk. Humans were built to squat, hinge, push, pull, twist, crawl, carry, and climb. Each pattern trains your fascia, balances your joints, and makes you resilient. If you only ever move one way, you'll eventually break.
- **Balance Your Work:** If your job is repetitive, your training should be the antidote. Desk worker? Open your chest, strengthen your back, mobilise your hips. Tradie swinging hammers? Build shoulder stability, train core endurance, stretch through the spine. Training should restore what work takes away.
- **Keep Fascia Fluid:** Fascia responds to load, movement, and variety. Walk daily. Do rotational stretches. Carry awkward weights. Bounce, jump, twist. If your training looks the same every week, your fascia stiffens. Keep it guessing, keep it flowing.
- **Respect the Pain Signal:** Don't fear pain — learn from it. Sharp, stabbing pain is a red light. Fatigue, burning, and mild soreness are orange lights. Controlled load in the "orange zone" is where adaptation happens. Training through pain recklessly makes things worse, but avoiding all discomfort keeps you fragile.
- **Daily Movement Is Non-Negotiable:** Strength training two or three times a week is essential, but it's not enough. Movement has to be part of your everyday life. Walk after meals. Stretch in work breaks. Take the stairs. Use your body every day, not just in one-hour gym sessions.

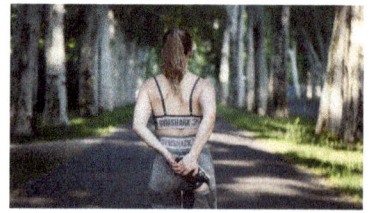

||| The Plan: Add It to Your Human Score

- **Undo Your Work Posture:** Do something that directly compensates for your daily workload. If you sit all day, stretch and mobilize your hips and back. If you're on your feet all day, elevate your legs, foam roll, and stretch. (1 point)
- **Strength Work:** Do at least 10 minutes of strength training using simple, functional movements — pushups, squats, pull-ups, or dumbbell presses. (1 point)
- **Daily Movement:** Accumulate at least 30 minutes of intentional movement (walking, training, playing, or sport). (1 point)

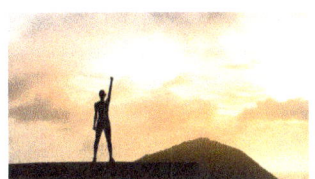

||| Final Word

Movement and strength is life. Muscles aren't for flexing in the mirror — they're the difference between standing tall and breaking down. Weakness means gravity and daily life wins. Strength means you win. It's not about six-packs or biceps. It's about whether your body is resilient enough to survive the demands of life. And for most people today, the answer is no.

Fascia stays fluid when you move. Joints stay young when you load them. Pain signals calm down when the body feels safe.

Weak humans break. Strong humans adapt and thrive.

So here's the blunt truth: every day you skip strength, you're letting yourself decay. Every time you move with intention, you're fighting back against gravity and time.

The choice is simple: build strength, or be broken by life.

||| References

1. Booth FW, Roberts CK, Laye MJ. Lack of exercise is a major cause of chronic diseases. Compr Physiol. 2012;2(2):1143–1211.
2. Frontera WR, Ochala J. Skeletal muscle: a brief review of structure and function. Calcif Tissue Int. 2015;96(3):183–195.
3. Rockson SG. Lymphedema. Am J Med. 2001;110(4):288–295.
4. Schleip R, et al. Fascia is able to contract in a smooth muscle-like manner and thereby influence musculoskeletal mechanics. Medical Hypotheses. 2005;65(2):273–277.
5. Chou R, et al. Diagnosis and treatment of low back pain: a joint clinical practice guideline. Ann Intern Med. 2007;147(7):478–491.
6. Landi F, et al. Sarcopenia as a risk factor for falls in elderly individuals: results from the ilSIRENTE study. Clin Nutr. 2012;31(5):652–658.
7. Narici MV, Maffulli N. Sarcopenia: characteristics, mechanisms and functional significance. Br Med Bull. 2010;95:139–159.
8. DeFronzo RA, et al. Insulin resistance: a multifaceted syndrome responsible for NIDDM, obesity, hypertension, dyslipidemia. Diabetes Care. 1991;14(3):173–194.
9. Guadalupe-Grau A, et al. Exercise and bone mass in adults. Sports Med. 2009;39(6):439–468.
10. Hayes LD, Elliott BT. Short-term exercise training improves testosterone, cortisol and health-related quality of life in aging men. Hormones. 2019;18(4):451–461.
11. Leong DP, et al. Prognostic value of grip strength: findings from the Prospective Urban Rural Epidemiology (PURE) study. Lancet. 2015;386(9990):266–273.

Chapter 6: Sleep & Recovery

The Forgotten Superpower

||| The Problem

Sleep has gone from being sacred to being optional. Modern culture glorifies the grind — late nights, early mornings, "I'll sleep when I'm dead." But that mindset is nothing to be proud of. Cutting sleep isn't strength, it's self-destruction. You're not showing discipline by running on fumes; you're slowly dismantling your body and mind.

The average adult today sleeps one to two hours less than people did a century ago [1]. Screens keep us up late, blasting our brains with artificial light at the exact time we should be producing melatonin. Blue light from phones, laptops, and TVs tricks your body into thinking it's still daytime, throwing your circadian rhythm completely out of sync [2]. "Add to that the constant presence of electrical devices near the bed — Wi-Fi routers, phones charging beside your head, even smart TVs left on standby — and your nervous system is never fully off-duty."

Work pressure, endless caffeine, alcohol before bed — they all chip away at the very thing our biology relies on to repair, recover, and stay alive. And people wonder why they're tired, overweight, anxious, foggy, inflamed, or depressed. Look around: society is sick, and one of the simplest reasons is staring us in the face. We've stopped respecting sleep.

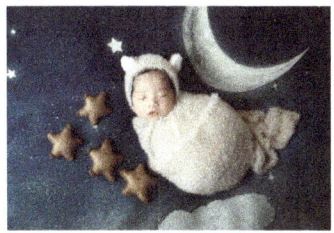

||| The Truth About Sleep

Sleep isn't downtime. It's the most powerful recovery tool you have. When you sleep, your body goes to work: repairing muscle, balancing hormones, sharpening memory, flushing toxins from the brain, and resetting the immune system [3,4].

The problem is most people don't respect it. They run on six hours, fuelled by caffeine, and wonder why they feel like crap. Poor sleep creeps in quietly but wrecks you deeply:

- **Just one night** of short sleep weakens your immune defence — natural killer cells (the immune system's first line of attack against viruses and abnormal cells) drop by up to 70% [5].
- **A week of 5–6 hours** a night makes your brain perform like you're legally drunk [6].
- **Chronic sleep loss** ramps up cortisol, slows metabolism, and raises the risk of weight gain, diabetes, heart disease, and depression [7,8].
- **Mentally, you're more reactive,** less resilient, and quicker to spiral. Lack of sleep is one of the strongest predictors of burnout and even suicidal thoughts [9].

That's the wake-up call. But here's the flip side: get sleep right, and the benefits are insane. Good sleep boosts testosterone [10], speeds recovery, clears your mind, lifts your mood, and sharpens focus. Just one solid night makes you feel more human; a week of consistent quality sleep can completely change how you look, move, and think.

Sleep is the ultimate multiplier. Every good choice you make — eating well, training, hydrating — works ten times better when your sleep backs it up.

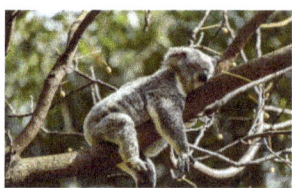

||| Recovery: The Forgotten Half of Progress

We live in a culture obsessed with the grind. Train harder. Work longer. Push through. But here's the truth — training, stress, and effort don't make you stronger. Recovery does.

Think about it: lifting weights doesn't make you stronger. It breaks muscle down. Strength comes from the repair that happens while you rest [11]. Same with learning, same with stress resilience. Stress is the signal; recovery is the adaptation. Without recovery, you just dig yourself deeper into fatigue, injury, and burnout.

And sleep is the ultimate anabolic state. No supplement, no drug, no hack even comes close to what eight solid hours can do for your body [12].

But recovery isn't just about sleep. It's also the little practices that downshift your nervous system, allowing you to recover and progress with training, work and life:

- **Breathwork:** Simple breathing techniques activate your parasympathetic nervous system — the body's natural "rest and digest" mode [13]. Slow, deep breaths calm your heart rate, lower stress hormones, and create instant grounding when life feels chaotic.
- **Meditation:** Stillness is medicine. Even 10 minutes a day helps lower cortisol, improve focus, and build mental resilience [14]. It's not about "clearing your mind" — it's about learning to control where your attention goes.
- **Naps:** A short 20–30 minute nap isn't laziness — it's a reset button. It recharges your energy, boosts alertness, and can even improve physical performance and creativity for the rest of the day [15].
- **Rest Days:** Muscles and tissues need time to rebuild. Active recovery — walking, stretching, or gentle movement — keeps blood flowing and joints lubricated while your body repairs the microdamage that training creates.
- **Cold & Heat Exposure:** Contrast therapy — like an ice bath or sauna — trains your body to handle stress. Cold exposure boosts circulation and resilience, while heat exposure improves recovery hormones and helps the body relax deeply afterward [16].

||| The Fix: How to Reclaim Your Sleep and Recovery

- **Morning Light:** Get sunlight within an hour of waking. It anchors your circadian rhythm, boosts serotonin (mood), and sets melatonin production for the night [17].
- **Darkness at Night:** Dim lights after sunset. Ditch screens at least 30 minutes before bed. If you must use devices, get blue-light filters or blue-blocking glasses. This one step alone can massively improve melatonin release [2].
- **Bedroom Setup:** Cool (around 18–20°C), dark (blackout curtains or eye mask), quiet (or white noise if needed). Your bedroom should feel like a cave. Keep electronics out of the room where possible. Phone in another room, Wi-Fi router off at night. Less stimulation, more deep sleep [18].
- **Consistency:** Go to bed and wake up at the same time every day, even weekends. Your body craves rhythm [19].
- **Caffeine Cut-Off:** No coffee or stimulants after midday. Caffeine has a half-life of 6+ hours — drink it late and you'll feel it at midnight [20].
- **Alcohol Reality Check:** Alcohol might knock you out, but it crushes REM sleep. Even small amounts fragment rest and leave you tired [21].
- **Wind-Down Ritual:** Breathwork, stretching, journaling, or reading. Signal to your body it's safe to power down [13,14].
- **Naps & Active Recovery:** Use short naps for a midday reset [15]. Use breathwork, meditation, and light movement to keep stress in check.
- **Respect Rest Days:** Recovery isn't laziness. It's part of the plan.
- **Track, Don't Depend:** Devices like smartwatches or sleep trackers can give short-term insight into patterns, but remember they're still electrical currents strapped to your body. Use them to learn, then minimise your reliance. True recovery comes from rhythm and habits, not data alone.

||| The Plan: Add It to Your Human Score

1. **8+ Hours of Quality Sleep:** Go to bed early enough to allow 8 hours of sleep. *(1 point)*
2. **Morning Light Before Screens:** Anchor your circadian rhythm by getting natural light before using devices. *(1 point)*
3. **Wind-Down Ritual:** Spend at least 30 minutes before bed with no screens, using breathwork, reading, or stretching instead. *(1 point)*

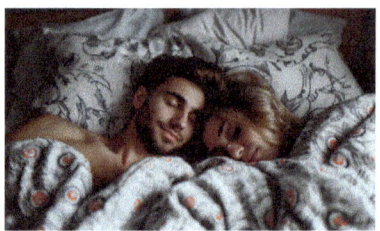

||| Final Word

Sleep is not wasted time. It's not weakness. It's the most powerful performance tool you have, and you're already wired for it.

You can eat perfectly, drink pure water, train hard, even meditate — but if you don't sleep, you're still broken. Every system in your body relies on it. Your brain, your hormones, your immune system, your mood, your strength — they all live or die by the quality of your sleep.

And here's the reality check: your body is not designed to recharge beside a glowing screen or a buzzing device. Sleep trackers, smart watches, Wi-Fi signals — they might help in the short term, but real recovery only happens when you allow your body to sink into darkness, silence, and rhythm.

So stop treating sleep like an afterthought. Respect it like oxygen, like food, like water. Build your nights around it. Guard it. Protect it.

Because here's the reality: the people walking around proud of their four-hour nights aren't superhuman. They're half-dead. And if you don't want to end up like them, you need to wake the f**k up to the power of sleep.

Close the laptop. Turn off the lights. Breathe. Rest. Recover. Sleep like a human.

||| References

1. National Sleep Foundation. (2015). Sleep duration recommendations. Sleep Health, 1(1), 40–43.
2. Cajochen, C., et al. (2011). Evening exposure to a light-emitting diodes (LED)-backlit computer screen affects circadian physiology. Journal of Applied Physiology, 110(5), 1432–1438.
3. Xie, L., et al. (2013). Sleep drives metabolite clearance from the adult brain. Science, 342(6156), 373–377.
4. Walker, M. (2017). Why We Sleep: Unlocking the Power of Sleep and Dreams. Scribner.
5. Irwin, M. R., et al. (1996). Partial night sleep deprivation reduces natural killer and cellular immune responses. FASEB Journal, 10(5), 643–653.
6. Williamson, A. M., & Feyer, A. M. (2000). Moderate sleep deprivation produces impairments in cognitive and motor performance equivalent to legally prescribed levels of alcohol intoxication. Occupational and Environmental Medicine, 57(10), 649–655.
7. Spiegel, K., et al. (1999). Impact of sleep debt on metabolic and endocrine function. The Lancet, 354(9188), 1435–1439.
8. Taheri, S., et al. (2004). Short sleep duration is associated with reduced leptin, elevated ghrelin, and increased body mass index. PLoS Medicine, 1(3), e62.
9. Bernert, R. A., et al. (2015). Sleep disturbances as an evidence-based suicide risk factor. Current Psychiatry Reports, 17(3), 554.
10. Leproult, R., & Van Cauter, E. (2011). Effect of sleep loss on neuroendocrine signals. Metabolism, 60(10), S11–S19.
11. Schoenfeld, B. J. (2010). The mechanisms of muscle hypertrophy and their application to resistance training. Journal of Strength and Conditioning Research, 24(10), 2857–2872.
12. Van Cauter, E., & Plat, L. (1996). Physiology of growth hormone secretion during sleep. Journal of Pediatrics, 128(5), S32–S37.
13. Brown, R. P., & Gerbarg, P. L. (2005). Sudarshan Kriya yogic breathing in the treatment of stress, anxiety, and depression. Journal of Alternative and Complementary Medicine, 11(4), 711–717.
14. Davidson, R. J., & McEwen, B. S. (2012). Social influences on neuroplasticity: stress and interventions to promote well-being. Nature Neuroscience, 15(5), 689–695.
15. Mednick, S. C., et al. (2003). Sleep-dependent learning: a nap is as good as a night. Nature Neuroscience, 6(7), 697–698.
16. Huttunen, P., et al. (2001). Health effects of cold exposure and sauna. International Journal of Circumpolar Health, 60(3), 422–429.
17. LeGates, T. A., et al. (2014). Circadian rhythms and mood: a review of the influence of light and the implications for treatment of mood disorders. Frontiers in Psychiatry, 5, 3.
18. Lan, L., et al. (2012). Thermal environment and sleep quality: a review. Energy and Buildings, 42(10), 1709–1716.
19. Monk, T. H., et al. (2003). Regularity of daily life in relation to personality, age, gender, sleep quality, and circadian rhythms. Journal of Sleep Research, 12(1), 63–70.
20. Drake, C., et al. (2013). Caffeine effects on sleep taken 0, 3, or 6 hours before going to bed. Journal of Clinical Sleep Medicine, 9(11), 1195–1200.
21. Ebrahim, I. O., et al. (2013). Alcohol and sleep I: effects on normal sleep. Alcoholism: Clinical and Experimental Research, 37(4), 539–549.

Chapter 7: Stress

Harnessing the Pressure

||| The Problem

Most people think of stress as something bad — the enemy. But stress itself isn't the problem. The real issue is that we either have too much of it, or not the right kind.

Stress is one of the most natural, essential parts of being human. It's your body's built-in defense mechanism, the alarm system that kept our ancestors alive. A predator appears? Stress gives you the speed to run. Food is scarce? Stress sharpens your focus to hunt. Stress was never meant to be constant — it was meant to come in short bursts to help us adapt and survive.

But modern life has turned stress into something it was never supposed to be. Instead of brief bursts of fight-or-flight, we live in low-grade, 24/7 stress. Traffic, bills, phones buzzing, deadlines, toxic food, lack of movement. Your body doesn't know the difference between a lion chasing you or an overdue mortgage notice — it reacts the same way. And when that system never switches off, it slowly destroys you.

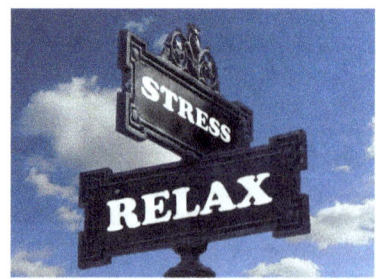

||| The Truth About Stress

Stress wears many faces. It shows up in three main forms:
- **Physical Stress:** the stress of movement (or lack of it). Exercise, injuries, repetitive work postures, sitting all day.
- **Chemical Stress:** toxins in food and water, alcohol, smoking, medications, pollution.
- **Emotional Stress:** thoughts, fears, trauma, relationships, finances, the stories we tell ourselves.

These stresses don't exist in isolation — they pile on top of each other. You can eat clean, but if your job is crushing you emotionally, you'll still get sick. You can meditate daily, but if you smoke a pack a day, your chemistry is still inflamed. The human body adds it all up.

Here's the thing most people miss: stress isn't just bad — it's necessary. Without stress, there is no growth. Muscles grow stronger under the stress of lifting weights. Bones become denser under the stress of impact. The immune system becomes sharper after facing stressors like heat, cold, or fasting [1]. And just like the body, the mind strengthens through challenge — every time you face fear, solve problems, or push through discomfort, your resilience expands and your capacity to handle life's pressures grows.

But here's where modern comforts ruin us: we've engineered most natural stress out of our lives. We never get too hot or too cold. We don't have to hunt or gather. We press a button and food arrives. We drive instead of walk. We wear cushioned shoes on flat floors. Life has become soft. And when life is too soft, humans become fragile.

Stress is the code written into your biology. The right amount builds resilience. Too little makes you weak. Too much breaks you down.

||| The Cost of Chronic Stress

When stress is unrelenting, your body never gets to reset. That's when stress becomes destructive.

- **Hormones hijacked:** Cortisol stays high, wrecking sleep, digestion, and recovery [2].
- **Constant Inflammation:** Chronic stress keeps the body inflamed, fueling joint pain, gut issues, heart disease, even cancers [3].
- **Immune system down:** Stress suppresses immunity, making you sick more often.
- **Mental burnout:** Anxiety, depression, mood swings, lack of focus [4].
- **Physical breakdown:** Chronic fatigue, muscle loss, weight gain, hormone imbalances.

It's not that stress is killing us. It's that the wrong kind of stress — constant, unresolved, modern stress — is.

||| The Fix: How to Master Stress

The goal isn't to eliminate stress. That's impossible. You will always have stress in your life. The goal is to train your brain and body to handle stress, so it doesn't seem like such a burden. Running a marathon is a huge physical stress on the body, but if you train for it, your body will be able to handle it and know how to recover from it.

1. Breathwork — Your Built-In Switch
Breathing is the fastest way to control your nervous system. Stress makes your breath shallow and rapid — your body thinks you're running from a threat. Deep, controlled breathing sends the opposite message: "I'm safe."

Why it works: Breath directly controls the vagus nerve, which governs heart rate, digestion, and relaxation. Slow, deep breathing lowers cortisol and adrenaline, shifting you from fight-or-flight into rest-and-digest [5].

Practical use:
- **Box breathing (inhale 4, hold 4, exhale 4, hold 4):** Calms the nervous system and sharpens focus.
- **Diaphragmatic breathing:** Place a hand on your belly. Breathe so the belly rises, not the chest. Do this for 5 minutes to lower stress hormones.
- **Breath holds:** After a calm inhale and exhale, hold your breath. Builds CO_2 tolerance and resilience to stress.

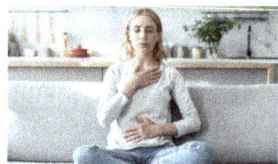

2. Seek Out Productive Stress
The body needs stress to stay strong. Without it, you become fragile. The key is controlled stress in short bursts — enough to challenge you, not to break you.

Why it works: Stress forces the body and mind to adapt, building strength, resilience, and recovery capacity. Without them, comfort slowly deconditions you [6].

Practical use:
- **Exercise:** Strength training or sprinting 2–3x per week. Builds muscle, bone density, and mental toughness.
- **Cold exposure:** 30–60 seconds in a cold shower. Teaches the nervous system to stay calm under stress.
- **Heat exposure:** Sauna sessions a few times per week. Trains cardiovascular resilience and aids detoxification.
- **Fasting:** Skip one meal occasionally. Sharpens insulin sensitivity and encourages cellular repair.

3. Move Daily

When stress hits, your body floods with hormones like adrenaline and cortisol. Perfect if you're escaping a predator — not so useful if you're sitting in traffic. If you don't move, those hormones linger, keeping you in a stressed state. Modern stress doesn't give you an outlet, so those hormones linger. Chronic high cortisol keeps blood sugar elevated, slows healing, and wrecks sleep [7].

Why it works: Movement "uses up" the fuel those hormones release. Exercise literally burns the sugar cortisol dumps into your blood, helping the nervous system reset back into balance.

Practical use:
- Walk for 10–15 minutes after stressful events (meetings, arguments, workdays).
- Add short stretch breaks during the day to release tension and lower cortisol.
- Use workouts as stress release valves — treat them as part of your recovery, not just fitness.

4. Disconnect — Step Away From the Noise

Phones, screens, and artificial lighting keep your nervous system wired on high alert. Every notification is a mini "fight-or-flight" trigger. Blue light at night tricks your brain into thinking it's still daytime, shutting down melatonin production and wrecking sleep [8].

Then there's light flicker — something most people don't even notice. LED and fluorescent lights flicker at high frequencies invisible to the eye, but your brain picks them up. This constant micro-stimulation keeps your nervous system buzzing and contributes to eye strain, headaches, and fatigue. It's like static you can't escape from.

Why it works: The brain evolved with natural cycles of light and dark, silence and sound. Disconnecting restores circadian rhythm, calms the nervous system, and lowers background stress your brain doesn't even realize it's carrying.

Practical use:
- Turn off devices for 1–2 hours before bed.
- Swap late-night screens for candles or warm incandescent bulbs.
- Use "digital breaks" — even 10 minutes of silence and no screens can reset your system.

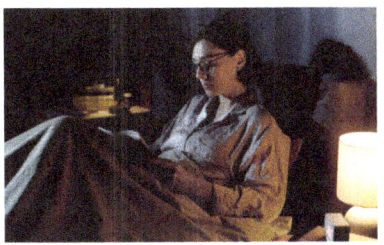

5. Reframe Your Stress
Not all stress is the same — what matters most is how you interpret it. Two people can face the same challenge: one breaks down, the other grows stronger. The difference? Perception.

Picture this: two people lose their job on the same day. One spirals — panic, self-doubt, sleepless nights. The other takes a breath, reassesses, and sees it as an opening to build something new. Same event. Two completely different physiological responses. One body floods with cortisol; the other releases adrenaline and focus. The difference isn't in what happened — it's in how it was perceived.

Why it works: Studies show that when people see stress as a challenge rather than a threat, their bodies release different hormonal profiles [9]. The stress response sharpens focus and energy without the same damaging effects.

Practical use:
- Before tough situations, tell yourself: "This is training, not punishment."
- When overwhelmed, reframe: "I'm being conditioned to handle more."
- Shift questions from "Why me?" to "What can I learn here?"

||| The Plan: Add It to Your Human Score

1. **Daily Breathwork Practice:** Spend 5–10 minutes focusing on your breath. Try slow nasal breathing, box breathing (inhale 4, hold 4, exhale 4, hold 4), Wim Hof method, or extended exhales to calm your nervous system. *(1 point)*
2. **Exposure to Natural Stressors:** Challenge your body with healthy stress — a cold shower, heat exposure (sauna, hot bath), or physical exercise. These stressors train resilience. *(1 point)*
3. **Conscious Downtime:** Disconnect daily from devices and artificial stimulation. Spend at least 15 minutes in stillness — meditation, time in nature, or simply sitting quietly. *(1 point)*

||| Final Word

Stress isn't a sign that something's wrong with you — it's proof that you're human. Feeling it doesn't mean you're weak, it means your body is doing what it was designed to do: protect, adapt, survive.

The real shift comes when you stop fearing stress and start working with it. With practice — through breath, movement, and a change in perspective — stress becomes less of a burden and more of a teacher. It shows you where you need to grow, and it gives you the fuel to get there.

Handled well, stress doesn't tear you down — it builds you up. It sharpens your edges, strengthens your core, and reminds you that you're far more capable than you think.

||| References

1. Mattson, M.P. (2014). Hormesis defined. Ageing Research Reviews.
2. Herbert, J. (2013). Cortisol and depression: three questions. Psychoneuroendocrinology.
3. Black, P.H., & Garbutt, L.D. (2002). Stress, inflammation and cardiovascular disease. Journal of Psychosomatic Research.
4. Segerstrom, S.C., & Miller, G.E. (2004). Psychological stress and the human immune system: meta-analytic study. Psychological Bulletin.
5. Jerath, R., et al. (2015). Physiology of long pranayamic breathing. Medical Hypotheses.
6. Lee, J., & Scott, S. (2011). Hormesis and human health. Dose-Response Journal.
7. Hackney, A.C. (2006). Stress and the neuroendocrine system: The role of exercise. Sports Medicine.
8. Cajochen, C., et al. (2011). Evening exposure to LED-backlit screens impacts melatonin secretion. Journal of Applied Physiology.
9. Crum, A.J., Salovey, P., & Achor, S. (2013). Rethinking stress: The role of mindsets. Journal of Personality and Social Psychology.

Chapter 8: ☠ Poison

Society's Accepted Toxins = Your Declining Health

||| The Problem

When you hear the word "poison," you probably picture a skull-and-crossbones bottle on a shelf — something obvious, something deadly in one hit. But the truth is, poison is everywhere, and most of us consume it daily. We pour it into glasses, light it on fire and inhale it, or eat it out of shiny packets with smiling cartoon characters on the front.

The real danger isn't that these poisons kill you instantly — it's that they drip-feed destruction into your body over years. Every cigarette, every drink, every dose of processed garbage forces your body to go into damage control. And while your body is busy fighting those toxins, it can't do the other things it's meant to do: heal injuries, repair cells, restore balance, and protect you from disease.

That's the trap: poison doesn't just make you feel rough the next morning. It robs you of your body's most powerful gift — its ability to heal. Instead of growing stronger from life's natural stressors — exercise, work, even daily wear and tear — your body stays stuck in survival mode, always fighting fires, never building resilience.

This is why poison is so dangerous: it doesn't just break you down directly. It stops you from repairing, recovering, and becoming the human you're supposed to be.

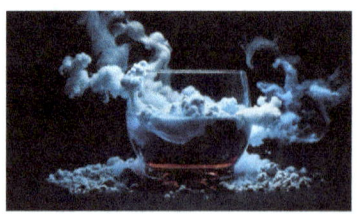

||| Alcohol — The Legal Toxin

Society dresses alcohol up as fun, social, and sophisticated. We toast with it at weddings, use it to unwind after work, and call it a reward for "getting through the week." But strip away the labels and marketing, and alcohol is just ethanol — a neurotoxin that damages the brain and body every single time you drink it [1].

Here's what really happens:
- **Liver:** Your liver treats alcohol as poison and drops everything to deal with it. While it's working overtime to detoxify ethanol, it can't properly process fat, hormones, or other toxins. This leads to fat storage, liver inflammation, and eventually fatty liver disease or cirrhosis [2]. Even small amounts add stress — the damage compounds over time.
- **Brain:** Alcohol slows down communication between brain cells by interfering with neurotransmitters like glutamate and GABA. In the short term, that means slurred speech, poor coordination, and bad decisions. Long term, alcohol literally shrinks brain tissue, reduces memory capacity, and increases risk of dementia, depression, and anxiety [3].
- **Hormones:** Alcohol disrupts the endocrine system. *In men,* testosterone production drops, leading to less muscle, lower sex drive, poor recovery, and even fertility issues [4]. *In women,* alcohol raises estrogen levels while reducing progesterone. This imbalance can fuel fat storage, disrupt menstrual cycles, worsen PMS, and increase risk of breast cancer.
- **Gut & Immune System:** Alcohol damages the gut lining, leading to leaky gut, inflammation, and disrupted microbiome. That disruption weakens the immune system, making you more vulnerable to illness and disease [5].
- **Sleep:** Many people use alcohol to "relax," but it doesn't create true rest. Alcohol sedates you, preventing deep REM and slow-wave sleep — the stages where your brain and body actually repair. You wake up inflamed, foggy, and unrestored, even if you slept a full night [6].

There's no dodging it: the World Health Organisation has made it clear that the healthiest amount of alcohol is zero [7]. Every drink is a dose of poison your body now has to fight off.

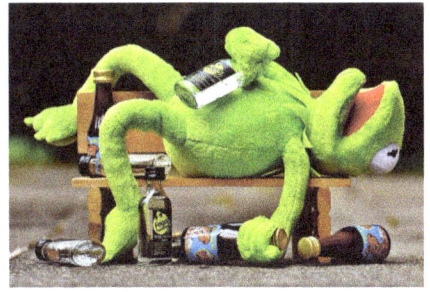

||| Smoking — Fire in the Lungs

A cigarette isn't just dried tobacco. It's a chemical cocktail — over 7,000 compounds, with at least 70 known to cause cancer [8]. When you light up, you're not just inhaling smoke — you're delivering poison directly into the bloodstream through the fastest gateway in the body: the lungs.

Here's what happens: The smoke is pulled deep into the alveoli — the tiny air sacs in your lungs where oxygen normally passes into your blood. Instead of clean oxygen, your bloodstream now absorbs carbon monoxide, tar, heavy metals, and toxic gases. Within seconds, those chemicals are circulating through every organ.

Some of the worst offenders:
- **Carbon monoxide:** Steals space from oxygen in your red blood cells, starving tissues of fuel. This is why smokers often feel tired, weak, and recover poorly.
- **Tar:** Sticky residue that coats the lungs, narrowing airways and trapping carcinogens in lung tissue. Over time, this leads to chronic bronchitis, emphysema, and lung cancer.
- **Formaldehyde:** The same chemical used to preserve dead bodies. It damages lung tissue and irritates the eyes, nose, and throat.
- **Arsenic:** A known poison and carcinogen — used in rat poison.
- **Cadmium:** A toxic heavy metal that damages the kidneys and weakens bones.
- **Benzene:** Found in gasoline. It damages bone marrow and increases leukemia risk [9].

The effects ripple out:
- **Lungs:** Air sacs break down, elasticity is lost, and breathing becomes harder (emphysema).
- **Circulation:** Blood vessels narrow, raising blood pressure and stroke risk. The heart works harder while getting less oxygen.
- **DNA damage:** Many of these chemicals directly damage DNA, creating mutations that lead to cancer. There's no "safe" amount — even one cigarette creates DNA changes [10].
- **Appearance:** Faster wrinkling, sagging skin, yellow teeth, and a distinct "smoker's face" from constant oxygen deprivation.

And the speed is shocking: within **10 seconds** of inhaling, nicotine hits the brain, flooding it with dopamine and hooking you to the cycle. The relief you feel from smoking isn't peace — it's the temporary end of withdrawal, bought at the cost of more damage [11].

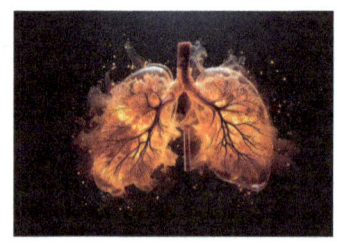

||| Hidden Poisons

Even if you don't drink or smoke, you're not in the clear. Poisons are hidden in plain sight — in the very things people eat and drink every single day.

- **Processed seed oils:** These cheap oils (canola, soybean, sunflower, corn) are heated, bleached, and deodorised before they ever hit your plate. By the time you cook with them, they're already oxidised. Once in your body, they trigger inflammation, damage cell membranes, and increase risk of heart disease and obesity [12].
- **Artificial sweeteners:** Marketed as "diet-friendly," but many disrupt the gut microbiome, confuse insulin responses, and can create the same sugar cravings they were meant to prevent [13]. Some, like aspartame, have been linked to headaches, mood changes, and neurological effects.
- **Preservatives & additives:** From sulphites in wine to nitrates in processed meats, these compounds extend shelf life at the expense of your cells. Some are directly linked to DNA damage and cancer risk [14].
- **Pesticides & herbicides:** Residues cling to non-organic fruits, vegetables, and grains. Over time, these chemicals can disrupt hormones, burden the liver, and weaken immunity [15].
- **Plastics:** Water bottles and food packaging leech microplastics and endocrine-disrupting chemicals like BPA into what you eat and drink. These act like fake hormones in your body, confusing your system and fueling problems like infertility, weight gain, and thyroid issues [16].

The real danger? None of these kill you instantly. They chip away quietly, day after day, leaving you tired, inflamed, overweight, and wondering why your body isn't working the way it should.

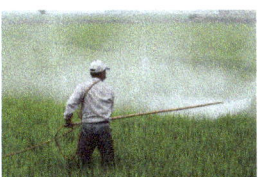

||| The Cost of Poison

Poison doesn't just damage one organ — it rewires your entire system. The price you pay is bigger than a hangover or a smoker's cough. Here's what's really happening:

- **Weaker immunity:** Alcohol, smoking, and chemical additives weaken your immune system's ability to respond to threats. White blood cells don't function properly, leaving you more vulnerable to infections, slower recovery from illness, and a higher risk of chronic disease.
- **Accelerated aging:** Poisons create oxidative stress — unstable molecules that damage cells and DNA [17]. This speeds up the aging process at every level: wrinkles on your skin, stiffness in your joints, and the slow breakdown of your organs.

- **Hormonal chaos:** Alcohol, smoking, and environmental toxins throw your endocrine system off balance. For men, testosterone crashes, leaving you weaker, heavier, and less driven. For women, elevated estrogen and reduced progesterone create irregular cycles, mood swings, PMS, weight gain, and higher risk of reproductive cancers.
- **Mental fog & mood disruption:** Nicotine, alcohol, and chemical additives disrupt neurotransmitters — the messengers of your brain. The result? Anxiety, depression, poor focus, and a constant rollercoaster of emotions. What feels like "relief" from drinking or smoking is just temporary numbing — the crash always follows.

You are what you consume. Your body is built cell by cell from what you put in it. Feed yourself poison, and you're building a body made of toxic bricks. That body won't stand strong. It will crack early, collapse under pressure, and fail to do what it was designed for: heal, adapt, and thrive

This doesn't stop with you. **Your choices ripple into the next generation.**

- **For women:** What you consume becomes the raw material your body uses to create life. Alcohol, nicotine, and toxins cross the placenta, shaping how a baby develops in the womb [18]. These poisons steal oxygen, nutrients, and stability from the very environment a child depends on to grow.

But it starts even earlier than that. A woman's health before pregnancy sets the stage for everything that follows. Years of alcohol, smoking, poor diet, and exposure to toxins don't just disappear once conception happens. They shape hormone balance, nutrient stores, egg quality, and the uterine environment. If the body is inflamed, nutrient-depleted, or stressed from years of poison, the baby's foundation is already compromised before it's even conceived.

A single choice at the dinner table or the bar becomes part of the child's foundation — brain, bones, organs, nervous system. Every mother wants to give their child the best start in life. Poison robs them of that.

- **For men:** The responsibility doesn't stop at the womb. Sperm doesn't just carry DNA — it carries epigenetic information. That means your choices as a man — alcohol, smoking, diet, stress — can literally switch genes on or off in your children before they're even conceived. Damaged sperm doesn't just lower fertility; it passes altered signals that can affect the health, resilience, and risks your kids face in life. Men who poison their bodies aren't just numbing themselves — they're programming weaknesses into the next generation.

This isn't about shame. It's about responsibility. It's about asking: What kind of foundation do you want your body — and your children's bodies — to be built on? If you want to leave behind strength, health, and resilience, it starts with removing poison today.

||| The Truth People Avoid

Deep down, everyone already knows alcohol and smoking are bad. No one lights a cigarette thinking it's a multivitamin, and no one wakes up after a night of drinking feeling "healthy." But people defend their poisons anyway, hiding behind excuses — "It's how I relax. Everyone does it. It's just part of life."

The truth is simple: these aren't harmless habits. They're slow-acting toxins that rob you of health, clarity, and time — keeping you stuck in cycles of fatigue and sickness while you convince yourself you're "fine."

You can't poison yourself and expect to be healthy. You can't smoke, drink, or eat chemical garbage and still hope for a strong body, a sharp mind, or a long life. You can't out-train it, out-supplement it, or meditate it away. What goes in becomes who you are.

The truth hurts, but it's supposed to. Sometimes the only way to wake up is to face the reality you've been avoiding — and finally stop defending what's been destroying you.

||| The Fix — How to Break Free

Breaking free isn't about being perfect — it's about being honest. Every step away from poison gives your body room to repair, rebuild, and breathe again.

- **Awareness:** The first step is calling poison what it is. Alcohol isn't "relaxation." Smoking isn't "just a habit." Processed junk isn't "food." The moment you strip away the excuses and see them for what they are — toxins breaking your body down — you take back control.
- **Replace rituals:** Humans love rituals. The drink after work, the smoke on a break, the snack in front of the TV. But those rituals don't have to disappear — they can be replaced. Swap alcohol for soda water with lime, kombucha, or herbal tea. Replace the cigarette hit with a few rounds of breathwork, a cold shower, or a quick burst of movement to give your brain the same dopamine kick without the destruction.
- **Detox lifestyle:** Once poison is reduced, give your body tools to clear the damage. Clean, unprocessed foods provide nutrients for repair. Filtered water eases the load on your liver and kidneys. Movement and sweating — through exercise, sauna, or even a brisk walk in the sun — flush toxins and reset your system. These aren't fads. They're the basics of how humans clean the house.
- **Change your circle:** Social pressure is one of the strongest poisons of all. If the people around you celebrate drinking, smoking, or eating garbage, you'll get dragged down with them. Surround yourself with people who value health and strength, and suddenly the hard choices become normal.
- **Progress, not perfection:** You don't need to quit everything overnight. Every skipped drink, every smoke you don't light, every cleaner meal is a win. Each choice lowers the toxic load and gives your body a better chance to heal. Progress compounds. Little by little, poison loses its grip.

||| The Plan: Add It to Your Human Score

1. **Alcohol-Free Day:** Consume zero alcohol today. Every alcohol-free day gives your body a chance to detoxify and your brain a chance to repair. *(1 point)*
2. **Smoke-Free Day:** No smoking or exposure to cigarette smoke. Your lungs, blood vessels, and energy levels recover even from one smoke-free day. *(1 point)*
3. **Avoid Hidden Poisons:** Skip one "socially accepted" toxin today — seed oils, artificial sweeteners, excess caffeine, or processed junk — and replace it with something nourishing and real. *(1 point)*

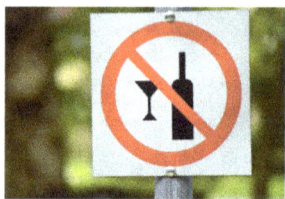

||| Final Word

Poison doesn't hit all at once. It steals life one drop at a time — a little less energy, a little less clarity, a little more breakdown. Most people don't notice until decades have passed and the damage is locked in.

But you don't have to live that story. Removing poison isn't about loss, it's about freedom. It's giving your body a chance to rebuild with real materials instead of toxic scraps.

Remember: you are what you consume. Feed yourself poison, and you'll live poisoned. Feed yourself life, and you'll live alive.

||| References

1. World Health Organization. (2018). Global status report on alcohol and health.
2. Rehm, J., et al. (2010). Alcohol consumption and liver cirrhosis. The Lancet.
3. Harper, C. (2009). The neurotoxicity of alcohol. Alcohol and Alcoholism.
4. Emanuele, M.A., & Emanuele, N.V. (1998). Alcohol's effects on male reproduction. Alcohol Health and Research World.
5. Barr, T., et al. (2016). Alcohol and the immune system. Alcohol Research: Current Reviews.
6. Ehlers, C.L., & Kupfer, D.J. (1989). Effects of ethanol on sleep. Advances in Alcohol & Substance Abuse.
7. WHO. (2023). No level of alcohol consumption is safe for our health.
8. U.S. Department of Health and Human Services. (2010). How Tobacco Smoke Causes Disease: The Biology and Behavioral Basis for Smoking-Attributable Disease.
9. Hecht, S.S. (2012). Research on tobacco carcinogenesis. Chemical Research in Toxicology.
10. Alexandrov, L.B., et al. (2016). Mutational signatures associated with tobacco smoking. Science.
11. Benowitz, N.L. (2010). Nicotine addiction. The New England Journal of Medicine.
12. Ramsden, C.E., et al. (2013). Dietary linoleic acid and inflammation. BMJ.
13. Suez, J., et al. (2014). Artificial sweeteners induce glucose intolerance by altering the gut microbiota. Nature.
14. Bouvard, V., et al. (2015). Carcinogenicity of consumption of red and processed meat. The Lancet Oncology.
15. Mnif, W., et al. (2011). Endocrine-disrupting pesticides. International Journal of Environmental Research and Public Health.
16. Gore, A.C., et al. (2015). Endocrine-disrupting chemicals: Effects on human health. Endocrine Reviews.
17. Liguori, I., et al. (2018). Oxidative stress and human diseases. Clinical Interventions in Aging.
18. Lange, S., et al. (2017). Alcohol use and pregnancy: a review. Reproductive Toxicology.

Chapter 9: Tribe & Connection

Alone We Break, Together We Thrive

||| The Problem

We live in the most connected time in history — phones buzzing, notifications flashing, thousands of "friends" online — and yet people are more alone than ever. Walk through a city and you'll see it: faces buried in screens, couples sitting together but not speaking, parents scrolling while their kids tug at their sleeves.

Loneliness isn't just "feeling sad." It's lethal. Studies show it's as bad for your health as smoking 15 cigarettes a day [1]. Divorce rates keep climbing. Rates of depression and anxiety are skyrocketing. Suicide has become one of the leading causes of death in young men [2]. And at the root of it all? Disconnection.

We've traded tribe for transactions. People spend more time chasing deadlines than nurturing relationships. Work comes first, family second — if at all. Parents are too exhausted or distracted to truly raise their kids, leaving children to be educated by TikTok, YouTube, and strangers online. Kids grow up without fathers to model strength and discipline, or without mothers to model care and stability. That absence leaves scars that ripple into adulthood.

Humans weren't designed for this. We're social, tribal animals. To strip connection out of life is to strip away one of the pillars of health.

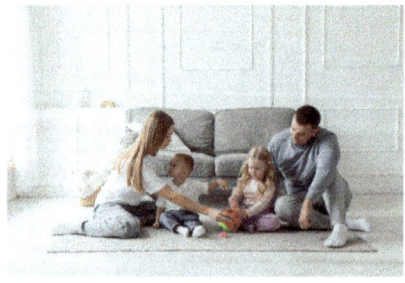

||| The Truth: We Are Tribal by Design

For millions of years, survival depended on tribe. Humans didn't make it to the top of the food chain because of sharp teeth or thick hides. We made it because we worked together. Men hunted, protected, and taught discipline. Women nurtured, gathered, and passed on wisdom. Children weren't raised by one set of exhausted parents — they were raised by the whole tribe. Connection wasn't optional; it was life itself.

That wiring hasn't changed. Your nervous system still looks for safety in groups, still regulates itself through eye contact, touch, and shared presence. Hormones like oxytocin and dopamine surge when you laugh, hug, or play with others [3]. Stress hormones drop when you feel supported. Even your immune system gets stronger when you belong to a group [4].

Look at children today. Play used to mean running with other kids, climbing trees, inventing games. Now it's iPads and isolation. Without connection, without role models of masculine strength and feminine care, kids grow up unsure of who they are or how to be. And adults aren't doing much better — numbed by work, dulled by screens, starved of community.

The truth is simple: you can eat clean, exercise daily, get sun and sleep, but if you're disconnected, you're still missing a fundamental human nutrient. Tribe is as essential as food, water, and oxygen. Without it, you don't just get lonely. You get sick.

||| The Cost of Disconnection

When tribe is stripped away, the body and mind pay the price.

- **Mental health collapse:** Disconnection drives anxiety, depression, and despair. In Australia, one in eight men will experience depression, and suicide remains the leading cause of death for men under 45 [2]. In the USA, loneliness has doubled in the past 50 years, with young people now the loneliest demographic [5]. These aren't statistics — they're signals that humans are starving for connection.
- **Stress overload:** Without a tribe, every burden falls on the individual. Bills, work, family pressures — all of it lands on one pair of shoulders. The nervous system was never designed for that. It was designed to share stress across a community. Alone, people drown.
- **Physical breakdown:** Loneliness increases inflammation, blood pressure, and the risk of heart disease [6]. One study found it carries the same mortality risk as obesity and smoking [1]. Chronic illness isn't just about food or movement — it's about whether you have people around you.
- **Generational wounds:** Kids raised without connection — without parents present, without extended family, without role models of strength and care — carry the weight into adulthood. Boys without fathers to model masculinity often grow unsure, lost, or angry. Girls without mothers present may struggle to develop trust, care, or self-worth. A disconnected generation raises an even more disconnected one.

The cost is everywhere. A society of soft, lonely, anxious humans who substitute real connection with virtual likes and scrolling feeds. Bodies breaking down, minds shutting off, kids growing up unanchored.

||| The Fix: Rebuilding Tribe in a Modern World

We can't go back to living in caves, but we can rebuild what matters most. Connection isn't about numbers — it's about depth. Here's where to start:

- **Prioritise real relationships:** Put family and close friends above work, above screens, above distractions. Have meals together. Share conversations without phones on the table. Laugh, argue, play — be human together.
- **Create modern tribes:** Gyms, sports clubs, men's groups, women's circles, community events — these are today's tribes. Find people who share values, who lift you up, who hold you accountable. Your nervous system doesn't care if the fire is digital or primal — it just needs to sit by it with others.
- **Play with your kids:** Children don't just need food and shelter. They need play, presence, and role models. Get on the floor with them. Teach them skills. Let them see strength and compassion in action. Every moment of connection is wiring their brain and shaping who they'll become.
- **Restore masculine and feminine roles:** Not rigid stereotypes — but balance. Kids thrive when they see men model discipline, strength, and protection, and women model care, empathy, and nurture. Both matter. Both are human. Missing one leaves a hole that kids will try to fill later in life, often in destructive ways.
- **Disconnect to reconnect:** Limit screen time. Replace endless scrolling with face-to-face time. Technology isn't evil, but it's a poor substitute for real presence. A hug, a look, a shared laugh — these are things no device can give.
- **Balance work with life:** Stop sacrificing family on the altar of your career. Work is necessary, but endless hours at the office or staring at emails won't hold your hand when you're sick, won't laugh with you at dinner, won't raise your kids to be strong. Time with family and tribe is the true wealth. Protect it like your health depends on it — because it does.

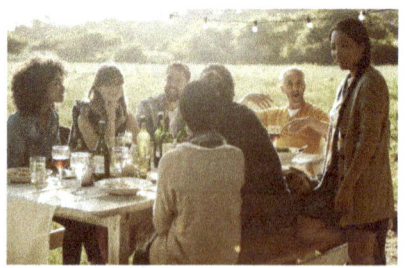

||| The Plan: Add It to Your Human Score

1. **Close Connection:** Spend meaningful, undistracted time with a close friend or family member — whether that's a chat, a meal, or shared activity. *(1 point)*
2. **Acts of Contribution:** Do one thing that benefits someone else — a small act of kindness, help, or support that strengthens your bond with others. *(1 point)*
3. **Community Connection:** Engage with your wider community daily. This could be joining in at the gym, playing sport, chatting with a neighbour, or even a positive interaction with a stranger. *(1 point)*

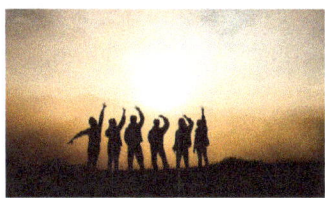

||| Final Word

Connection is not optional. It's not a "nice to have." It's as essential as water, sunlight, and food. Without it, you will wither — mentally, physically, spiritually.

We've been tricked into thinking independence is the highest goal. But humans aren't built to be independent. We're built to be interdependent. To lean on each other. To raise children together. To share the load of life.

The truth is, you can lift weights, eat clean, get sun, and sleep deeply, but if you're doing it all alone, you'll still feel empty. Tribe is the missing nutrient. Rebuild it, and you'll feel a kind of strength no supplement or workout can give.

And stop pretending work will make up for it. No paycheck, promotion, or deadline is worth more than the time you spend with the people who love you. In the end, no one remembers the hours you billed or the titles you held. They remember how present you were.

When you reconnect with others, you reconnect with yourself. And that is what makes us truly human.

||| References

1. Holt-Lunstad, J., et al. (2010). Social relationships and mortality risk: A meta-analytic review. PLoS Medicine.
2. Australian Bureau of Statistics (2022). Causes of Death, Australia.
3. Carter, C.S. (2014). Oxytocin pathways and the evolution of human behavior. Annual Review of Psychology.
4. Cole, S.W. (2009). Social regulation of human gene expression: mechanisms and implications. American Journal of Public Health.
5. Twenge, J.M., et al. (2019). Age, period, and cohort trends in loneliness among US adolescents and young adults. Journal of Social and Personal Relationships.
6. Hawkley, L.C., & Cacioppo, J.T. (2010). Loneliness matters: a theoretical and empirical review. Annals of Behavioral Medicine.

Chapter 10: Spirit, Energy & Thoughts

Beyond the Physical

||| The Problem

Most people think of themselves as a physical body — skin, muscle, bone, organs. That's what the eye sees, so that's where most stop. But this picture is incomplete. It leaves out the very thing that makes life possible.

The body you live in feels solid and permanent, but physics tells a different story. Beneath the surface, every cell and structure is built from atoms, and atoms themselves are nearly all empty space. What gives them shape is not solidity, but movement — energy vibrating and organising itself into the patterns we recognise as the physical world.

Yet modern culture rarely talks about this. We reduce humans to mechanical systems: calories in, calories out; symptoms and pills; flesh that wears out over time. That limited view ignores the most fundamental fact of existence — that at our core, we are **energy**, constantly vibrating, interacting, and exchanging with the world around us.

When you forget this, you misunderstand health itself. Because health isn't just about muscles, joints, or organs — it's about the flow and direction of energy that shapes every one of those parts.

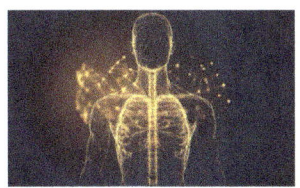

||| The Truth: Everything Is Energy

At the most basic level, the human body — and everything around it — is built from atoms. Atoms are not solid units. They are more than 99% empty space, with a dense nucleus surrounded by electrons in constant motion. What we perceive as solid matter is, in reality, patterns of vibration and force [1].

This applies universally. The same building blocks that form your body also form the chair you sit on, the air you breathe, and the light that reaches your eyes. The difference lies in the frequency and organisation of the vibrations:

- **Sound:** Pressure waves moving through air that your ears translate into meaning.
- **Light:** Vibrations in the electromagnetic spectrum, interpreted by your eyes as colour.
- **Air:** A constant ocean of unseen particles flowing through you with every breath
- **Thoughts:** Invisible frequencies pulsing through the brain — sparks of energy that don't just stay in your head, but echo through your body and the space around you.

Seen from this perspective, nothing in the world is truly separate. Everything is part of a continuous field of energy, and human beings are not observers standing outside of it — we are embedded within it, shaped by it, and constantly influencing it.

Modern science supports this view. Psychoneuroimmunology demonstrates how mental states such as stress directly alter immune function [2]. Epigenetics shows that environment and thought patterns can influence gene expression over time [3]. Neurocardiology reveals how heart rhythms affect brain function and emotional regulation [4].

The implication is simple: health and human experience cannot be reduced to mechanical parts alone. They are the result of how energy is generated, directed, and integrated throughout the body and mind. Recognising this is the first step toward understanding what it truly means to be human.

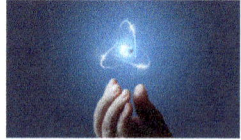

||| Thoughts as Energy

Thoughts are not harmless chatter. They are real, physical events that ripple through your entire body.

Every time you think, neurons in your brain fire tiny electrical charges. Those charges release chemicals — hormones, neurotransmitters — that flood your body and shift how you feel. A positive thought can lift your chest, calm your heart, and relax your gut. A negative one can tighten your muscles, raise your blood pressure, and flood your bloodstream with cortisol.

Over time, repeated thoughts carve grooves in the nervous system — habits of energy that shape your biology. These mental patterns don't just live in your head; they alter your hormones, immune function, and even gene expression [5].

Every thought sends a ripple through your body's chemistry, influencing how you feel, how you heal, and ultimately, how long you live. The story you repeat in your mind becomes the biology you live in.

That's the power of thought energy. It's not mystical. It's practical biology. What you think shapes who you are.

||| Perception Shapes Reality

The world doesn't come to you as raw data. It comes filtered. Every sound, colour, word, and experience passes through the lens of your nervous system before you ever become aware of it. That lens is shaped by memory, belief, and expectation. In other words, you don't just experience reality — you interpret it.

Two people can live through the same event and walk away with entirely different stories. One sees loss, the other sees opportunity. One feels broken, the other feels challenged. The difference isn't in the event itself but in the perception applied to it.

Imagine two people lose their job on the same day. One spirals: "I'm worthless, I'll never recover," and sinks into depression. The other reframes: "This is my chance to start fresh, to build something better," and uses it as fuel. The event is identical. The outcomes couldn't be further apart. What changed wasn't the circumstance — it was perception.

Neuroscience confirms this. The brain is constantly predicting and filling in the gaps of reality. What you perceive as "truth" is in many ways a construction — a best guess — based on past experiences and what your brain expects to find. This isn't weakness; it's efficiency. But it means perception carries enormous power.

Perception influences chemistry. A threat perceived — even if imagined — raises cortisol, tightens muscles, and accelerates the heart. Safety perceived — even if the external situation hasn't changed — lowers stress hormones, steadies the pulse, and calms the mind. Over time, these repeated responses condition the body into states of health or states of disease.

This is why shifting perspective can feel like shifting worlds. The event may not change, but your biology does. When you learn to reframe — to see possibility instead of limitation, growth instead of loss — your body responds differently. Hormones rebalance, immunity steadies, energy returns. Perception isn't abstract; it's a biological switch that shapes how you live.

||| Negative Energy & Stored Stress

Emotions are not just passing feelings in your head. They are full-body events. Every emotion has a physiological footprint: hormones are released, muscles tense or relax, breathing changes, heart rate shifts. When emotions move through and resolve, the body resets. But when they are suppressed, ignored, or repeated without release, the body doesn't forget — it stores them.

Trauma is the clearest example: unresolved survival energy shows up as persistent tension, protective postures, and pain without a single mechanical cause. Over time, chronic stress loads immunity, gut function, and pain pathways [6,7]. Clinically, unless that stored energy is acknowledged and released, the pattern tends to resurface.

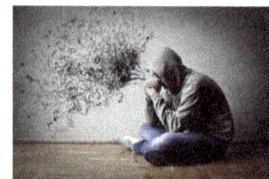

You can see it in people's bodies. Grief slumps the shoulders forward and caves the chest in, as if the body is literally protecting the heart. Anger clenches the jaw, tightens the fists, and pulls the shoulders up toward the ears. Anxiety lives in restless legs, fidgeting hands, shallow breaths, and a tight gut. Over years, these postures and patterns don't just signal emotion — they become the body's default state.

Science is beginning to catch up with what healers have seen for centuries. Chronic stress and unresolved emotion are linked to autoimmune disease, digestive disorders, and persistent pain syndromes. These aren't metaphors — they're nervous system memories embedded into tissue.

As a chiropractor, I see it daily. Patients come in with "physical pain," but the scans and exams don't explain the severity. Their body is carrying something more — years of unprocessed stress layered into posture, muscle tone, and movement patterns. You can adjust the spine, stretch the muscles, strengthen the core — but unless the emotional energy is acknowledged and released, the problem resurfaces.

The reality is simple: negative energy doesn't vanish just because you try to ignore it. It either moves through you, or it gets stored in you. And over time, stored energy shapes not just how you feel, but how your body functions — down to the level of immunity, hormones, and healing.

60

||| External Influences: Hijacking the Mind

Your thoughts don't form in isolation. They are constantly shaped by what you consume. News cycles, advertising, social media feeds, television, even casual conversations — all of these provide inputs that your brain uses to construct its version of reality.

The human brain is programmable. Repetition wires belief. Hear something often enough — whether it's "you're not good enough," "buy this to be happy," or "the world is dangerous" — and over time it becomes the filter through which you see life. The content doesn't need to be true; it only needs to be consistent.

Modern inputs are designed for this. Social media platforms run on dopamine loops — each like, scroll, or notification is engineered to keep you hooked. News thrives on fear and outrage because those emotions grab attention faster than calm or nuance. Advertising is built on comparison, making you feel like you're always lacking something unless you buy more. These aren't accidents; they're strategies.

Biologically, the effects are clear. Constant exposure to fear-based media elevates cortisol and keeps the nervous system in a low-level fight-or-flight state. Endless scrolling hijacks dopamine cycles, leaving people restless, unfocused, and unable to feel satisfied with simple experiences. Comparison erodes self-worth and creates chronic stress, which over time disrupts hormones, sleep, and immunity.

And here's the part most people don't want to admit: your mind is not fully your own. The beliefs you hold, the things you worry about, even what you desire — much of it has been planted there by external forces. If you don't consciously choose what you allow in, you become a passenger in your own life, running programs that were written by corporations, media outlets, and algorithms.

Regaining sovereignty of thought is not optional if you want health, clarity, and freedom. You cannot build a strong, resilient body while your mind is being hijacked. Taking back control means becoming intentional about what you consume, who you listen to, and where your attention goes. Because in the end, attention is energy — and if you don't direct it, someone else will.

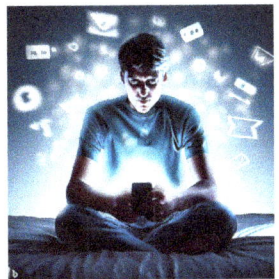

||| The Fix: Reclaiming Spirit & Thought Energy

Reclaiming your energy isn't about chasing mystical experiences or learning complicated rituals. It starts with small, deliberate choices that bring your mind back under your control and remind your body what balance feels like.

Awareness
The first step is simply noticing. Most people run on autopilot, unaware of the constant stream of thoughts moving through their head. But thoughts lose power the moment you observe them. Practices like journaling, mindfulness, or simply pausing to ask, "what am I thinking right now?" shift you from being the thought to being the observer of it. That small gap is where choice returns.

Reframing
Once awareness is in place, the next step is reframing. Life will throw challenges, but perception decides whether those challenges become trauma or growth. Reframing isn't denial; it's choosing a different interpretation. Losing a job can be the end of security or the start of freedom. An argument with a partner can be proof of distance or an invitation to connect differently. Each frame carries a different energetic and biological response — one closes the body down, the other opens it up.

Breathwork & Meditation
Breath is the fastest way to change your state. Slow, controlled breathing lowers cortisol, steadies the heart, and rebalances the nervous system in minutes. Meditation extends that effect, training the brain to step out of constant reactivity and into calm observation. These aren't abstract practices; they're biological resets. A few minutes of breathwork or meditation daily is enough to shift how the body processes stress and how the mind processes thought.

Spiritual Practice
Connection to something larger than yourself is a fundamental human need. It doesn't matter whether you call it God, nature, or simply the order of the universe. What matters is making time for it. That might mean prayer, gratitude, walking in silence outdoors, or simply sitting still and remembering you are part of something bigger. These practices recalibrate perspective, soften ego, and bring coherence to the energy you project into the world.

Protecting Inputs
Your energy reflects what you feed it. Constant negativity, endless scrolling, and fear-based news will keep your biology on edge. Choosing your inputs carefully — books that inspire, conversations that nourish, environments that calm — isn't avoidance, it's hygiene. Just as you wouldn't drink polluted water and expect to stay healthy, you can't consume polluted information and expect a clear mind. Protect your attention as fiercely as you protect your body, because both are shaped by what you allow in.

The practices are simple, but the effects are profound. Bit by bit, these choices train the body and mind to reset. They redirect energy from chaos into order, from fragmentation into clarity. And when energy is ordered, the rest of health follows.

||| The Plan: Add It to Your Human Score

1. **Awareness of Thought Patterns:** Take notice throughout the day when your mind drifts into negativity, stress, or self-criticism. Simply catching yourself is the first step toward change. *(1 point)*
2. **Reframe Every Negative Thought:** Each time you notice a negative thought, actively replace it with a positive or empowering perspective. Don't just let it pass — redirect it. *(1 point)*
3. **Eliminate Negative Inputs:** Reduce or remove one source of negativity in your life today — whether it's doom-scrolling the news, following toxic people on social media, or engaging with people who drain you. *(1 point)*

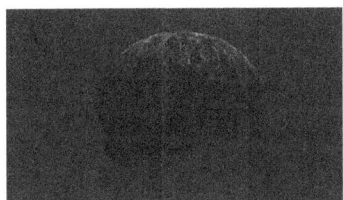

||| Final Word

You are not just a body moving through the world — you are energy in motion, alive in every breath, every thought, every connection. The patterns you create inside yourself shape the life you experience outside yourself. That means you are never stuck. At any moment, you can redirect your energy toward healing, clarity, and strength.

Your thoughts are not chains. They are tools. With awareness, with breath, with intention, you can change the way you feel, the way you see, and the way you live. You are capable of creating calm where there was chaos, joy where there was numbness, and health where there was decline.

This is not about perfection — it's about presence. When you begin to see yourself as energy, you start to see the beauty in being human again. You can choose to align with vitality, with connection, with gratitude. And in that choice, life becomes lighter, fuller, and worth loving.

||| References

1. Feynman, R. The Feynman Lectures on Physics, Vol. I–III. Addison-Wesley. (Atomic structure; scale and "empty space").
2. Ader, R. (2001). Psychoneuroimmunology. Current Directions in Psychological Science, 10(3), 94–98.
3. Weaver, I.C.G., et al. (2004). Epigenetic programming by maternal behavior. Nature Neuroscience, 7, 847–854.
4. Thayer, J.F., Åhs, F., Fredrikson, M., Sollers, J.J., & Wager, T.D. (2012). A meta-analysis of HRV and neuroimaging: implications for emotion regulation and health. Neuroscience & Biobehavioral Reviews, 36(2), 747–756.
5. Kaliman, P., et al. (2014). Rapid changes in histone deacetylases and inflammatory gene expression after a day of mindfulness practice. Psychoneuroendocrinology, 40, 96–107.
6. Cohen, S., Janicki-Deverts, D., & Miller, G.E. (2007/2012). Psychological stress and disease. JAMA / Annual Review of Psychology.
7. van der Kolk, B. (2014). The Body Keeps the Score. Viking. (Clinical synthesis on trauma's bodily imprint.)

Becoming Human Again

Stop. Take a breath. Look at your life. Ask yourself — how human are you, really?

You weren't built to sit, scroll, stress, and numb yourself through each day. You were built to rise with the sun, drink clean water, move with strength, eat real food, sleep deeply, and connect with your tribe. That's how humans survived and thrived for millions of years. That's still what makes you alive today.

The modern world isn't the enemy — but it will turn you into a robot if you let it. Technology and work can either steal your humanity or support it. Use the tools, don't let them use you. Let them help you move, breathe, rest, and connect — not distract you from being alive.

And yes, life makes it hard sometimes. Shift work, long hours, stress — not everyone can live perfectly in rhythm with nature. But you can still choose. Do what you can today. Then a little more tomorrow. Each choice brings you closer to strength, clarity, and freedom.

You don't need to be perfect — you just need to begin. Step by step, point by point, you'll reconnect with the basics that always worked.

Remember, you are human. You are a part of the earth. Modern society has just disconnected us more than it should have. So now it's time to take your life back. To recreate the unlimited energy within you, and become the best version of yourself that you never thought was possible.

It's time to become *HUMAN AGAIN*.

||| How to Use Your Human Score

This score isn't about perfection — it's about awareness and consistency. Each day, go through the checklist and give yourself 1 point for every habit you complete. At the end of the day, tally your score. At the end of the week, total all 7 days to see your weekly score.

Think of it like this: every point is a win for your body, mind, and soul. Some days you'll crush it, other days life will get in the way — and that's fine. The goal isn't 100%, the goal is progress. Over time, these daily wins stack up into lasting strength, clarity, and resilience.

Print the table, fill it in daily, and watch your human score climb. The higher your score, the closer you are to living the way humans were designed to live.

||| Human Score Grading Scale

Daily Grading (out of 30)
- **0–10 points** → Needs Work (your body is running on empty)
- **11–20 points** → Solid Foundation (you're building momentum, keep stacking habits)
- **21–25 points** → Strong Human (you're thriving in most areas, refine the weak spots)
- **26–30 points** → Optimal Human (you're living in alignment, few modern humans ever get here consistently)

||| Weekly Grading (out of 210)

- **0–70 points** → Needs Work (modern life has pulled you far from your potential)
- **71–140 points** → Solid Foundation (you're making progress, your systems are responding)
- **141–180 points** → Strong Human (your lifestyle supports health and resilience most of the time)
- **181–210 points** → Optimal Human (you're living in full alignment — this is rare, but it's the benchmark to strive for)

	Tasks	Mon	Tue	Wed	Thu	Fri	Sat	Sun
Sun	**Morning Sunlight:** Get at least 10 minutes of natural sunlight on your skin and eyes within the first hour of waking. No sunglasses. *(1 point)* **Midday Exposure:** Expose as much skin as possible to the midday sun for 10–20 minutes, depending on your skin type and tolerance. *(1 point)* **Minimal Sunglasses Use:** Only wear sunglasses when glare is unbearable. Let your eyes take in natural light to keep your circadian rhythm sharp. *(1 point)*							
Earthing	**Daily Barefoot Time:** Spend at least 10 minutes with bare skin touching natural ground (grass, dirt, sand, soil). *(1 point)* **Flat Shoes, Not Heels:** Wear flat-soled shoes (zero or minimal heel lift) throughout the day. Minimalist shoes are ideal, but the main rule is *no elevated heels*. *(1 point)* **Strengthen the Feet:** Do one drill to build foot strength and alignment — tip-toe walking, toe spacers, towel scrunches, or barefoot balance work. *(1 point)*							
Water	**Filtered Water (all day):** Ditch the tap water and drink filtered water throughout the day. Every sip supports your cells instead of drowning them in chemicals. *(1 point)* **Electrolyte Support (once daily):** Add a pinch of natural sea salt/celtic salt, trace minerals, or electrolytes once a day to restore what sweat, stress, and caffeine drain from your system. *(1 point)* **Plastic-Free (glass/steel only):** Switch to glass or stainless steel for both storage and drinking. It's a small shift that keeps your water — and your body — clean. *(1 point)*							
Food	**Eat Real Food (meat, fruit, vegetables):** Every meal today comes from nature. If it grew in the ground, fell from a tree, or walked the earth, it counts. *(1 point)* **Zero Processed Foods:** No bread, no soft drinks, no packaged "food-like" products. If it came with a barcode or a long list of ingredients, skip it. *(1 point)* **Conscious Eating:** Sit down, slow down, and treat eating as a ritual. No scrolling, no TV, no distractions — just you, your food, and the purpose of fueling your body. *(1 point)*							
Strength & Movement	**Undo Your Work Posture:** Do something that directly compensates for your daily workload. If you sit all day, stretch and mobilize your hips and back. If you're on your feet all day, elevate your legs, foam roll, and stretch. *(1 point)* **Strength Work:** Do at least 10 minutes of strength training using simple, functional movements — pushups, squats, pull-ups, or dumbbell presses. *(1 point)* **Daily Movement:** Accumulate at least 30 minutes of intentional movement (walking, training, playing, or sport). *(1 point)*							
Sleep	**8+ Hours of Quality Sleep:** Go to bed early enough to allow 8 hours of sleep. *(1 point)* **Morning Light Before Screens:** Anchor your circadian rhythm by getting natural light before using devices. *(1 point)* **Wind-Down Ritual:** Spend at least 30 minutes before bed with no screens, using breathwork, reading, or stretching instead. *(1 point)*							

	Tasks	Mon	Tue	Wed	Thu	Fri	Sat	Sun
Stress	**Daily Breathwork Practice:** Spend 5–10 minutes focusing on your breath. Try slow nasal breathing, box breathing (inhale 4, hold 4, exhale 4, hold 4), Wim Hof method, or extended exhales to calm your nervous system. *(1 point)* **Exposure to Natural Stressors:** Challenge your body with healthy stress — a cold shower, heat exposure (sauna, hot bath), or physical exercise. These stressors train resilience. *(1 point)* **Conscious Downtime:** Disconnect daily from devices and artificial stimulation. Spend at least 15 minutes in stillness — meditation, time in nature, or simply sitting quietly. *(1 point)*							
Poison	**Alcohol-Free Day:** Consume zero alcohol today. Every alcohol-free day gives your body a chance to detoxify and your brain a chance to repair. *(1 point)* **Smoke-Free Day:** No smoking or exposure to cigarette smoke. Your lungs, blood vessels, and energy levels recover even from one smoke-free day. *(1 point)* **Avoid Hidden Poisons:** Skip one "socially accepted" toxin today — seed oils, artificial sweeteners, excess caffeine, or processed junk — and replace it with something nourishing and real. *(1 point)*							
Tribe	**Close Connection:** Spend meaningful, undistracted time with a close friend or family member — whether that's a chat, a meal, or shared activity. *(1 point)* **Acts of Contribution:** Do one thing that benefits someone else — a small act of kindness, help, or support that strengthens your bond with others. *(1 point)* **Community Connection:** Engage with your wider community daily. This could be joining in at the gym, playing sport, chatting with a neighbour, or even a positive interaction with a stranger. *(1 point)*							
Thoughts	**Awareness of Thought Patterns:** Take notice throughout the day when your mind drifts into negativity, stress, or self-criticism. Simply catching yourself is the first step toward change. *(1 point)* **Reframe Every Negative Thought:** Each time you notice a negative thought, actively replace it with a positive or empowering perspective. Don't just let it pass — redirect it. *(1 point)* **Eliminate Negative Inputs:** Reduce or remove one source of negativity in your life today — whether it's doom-scrolling the news, following toxic people on social media, or engaging with people who drain you. *(1 point)*							
	Total Daily Score (30)							
	Total Weekly Score (210)							